QM Medical Libraries

24 1007182 8

BARTS AND THE LONDON LIBRARY

OXFORD HANDBOOKS IN EMERGENCY MEDICINE

BARTS AND THE LONDON
SCHOOL OF MEDICINE AND DENTISTRY
WHITECHAPEL LIBRARY,TURNER STREET, LONDON E1 2AD
020 7882 7110

ONE WEEK LOAN
Book are to be returned on or before the last date below,
otherwise fines may be charged.

- 2 FEB 2006

2 0 FEB 2006

- 9 NOV 2007

on)

16. Cardiopulmonary Resuscitation (second edition)
DAVID V. SKINNER AND RICHARD VINCENT

17. Emergency Management of Hand Injuries
G. R. WILSON, P. A. NEE, AND J. S. WATSON

18. Musculo-skeletal Problems in Emergency Medicine
JIM WARDROPE AND BRYAN ENGLISH

19. Anaesthesia and A   e
(second edition)
KAREN A. ILLINGWO

D1380708

This series has already established itself as the essential reference series for staff in A & E departments.

Each book begins with an introduction to the topic, including epidemiology where appropriate. The clinical presentation and the immediate practical management of common conditions are described in detail, enabling the casualty officer or nurse to deal with the problem on the spot. Where appropriate a specific course of action is recommended for each situation and alternatives discussed. Information is clearly laid out and easy to find — important for situations where swift action may be vital.

Details on when, how, and to whom to refer patients are covered, as well as the information required at referral, and what this information is used for. The management of the patient after referral to a specialist is also outlined.

The next of each book is supplemented with checklists, key points, clear diagrams illustrating practical procedures, and recommendations for further reading.

The Oxford Handbooks in Emergency Medicine are an invaluable resource for every member of the A & E team, written and edited by clinicians at the sharp end.

Musculo-skeletal problems in emergency medicine

Jim Wardrope
Consultant in Accident and Emergency Medicine,
Northern General Hospital,
Sheffield

and

Bryan English
Consultant Orthopaedic Physician,
Northern General Hospital,
Sheffield

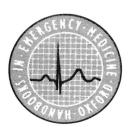

OXFORD UNIVERSITY PRESS

*This book has been printed digitally and produced in a standard specification
in order to ensure its continuing availability*

OXFORD
UNIVERSITY PRESS

Great Clarendon Street, Oxford OX2 6DP

Oxford University Press is a department of the University of Oxford.
It furthers the University@ objective of excellence in research, scholarship,
and education by publishing worldwide in

Oxford New York

Auckland Bangkok Buenos Aires Cape Town Chennai
Dar es Salaam Delhi Hong Kong Istanbul Karachi Kolkata
Kuala Lumpur Madrid Melbourne Mexico City Mumbai Nairobi
S‹o Paulo Shanghai Taipei Tokyo Toronto

Oxford is a registered trade mark of Oxford University Press
in the UK and in certain other countries

Published in the United States
by Oxford University Press Inc., New York

© Jim Wardrope and Bryan English 1998

The moral rights of the author have been asserted

Database right Oxford University Press (maker)

Reprinted 2003

All rights reserved. No part of this publication may be reproduced,
stored in a retrieval system, or transmitted, in any form or by any means,
without the prior permission in writing of Oxford University Press,
or as expressly permitted by law, or under terms agreed with the appropriate
reprographics rights organization. Enquiries concerning reproduction
outside the scope of the above should be sent to the Rights Department,
Oxford University Press, at the address above

You must not circulate this book in any other binding or cover
and you must impose this same condition on any acquirer

ISBN 0-19-262862-3

Printed in Great Britain by
Antony Rowe Ltd., Eastbourne

SBRLSMD

CLASS MARK	WB105 WAR
CIRC TYPE	1 WK
SUPPLIER	CIS- £33.45 30110 4
READING LIST	
OLD ED CHECK	

Preface

What is a sprained ankle? How is it treated? Could the ankle pain be due to osteomyelitis? Common problems in A&E medicine with an estimated 3 million attendances each year are due to musculo-skeletal problems. This work is not as high profile as resuscitation or the care of serious injury, but it is the area where statistically A&E doctors are most likely to make an error. The misdiagnosis of a septic arthritis is as potentially lethal as missing an extradural haemorrhage.

How to use this book

The whole emphasis of the book is on the *diagnosis* of acute musculo-skeletal problems. Chapter 2 is the key to understanding the system of assessment used throughout the book. Reading, *practising*, and understanding the techniques and 'language' of examination is recommended as an essential starting point.

The regional chapters all have a similar structure beginning with anatomy and the examination. The rest of each chapter is structured around the *clinical presentations* (see list p. 0). Patients come to A&E not with a diagnosis but with a major presenting symptom, for example knee pain after an injury or a limping child with no history of injury.

The book emphasizes the distinction between patients with an acute traumatic injury (90 per cent of workload) and those with no history of trauma (where the diagnosis is often difficult). Since many of the non-traumatic problems are rare they are highlighted so that at least they might be *considered*.

The system of assessment follows standard practice, but the investigation, treatment, and follow-up may vary between departments. Many of the common problems will be well described in local guidelines.

Sheffield   J. W.
October 1997   B. E.

Acknowledgements

This book is a synthesis of musculo-skeletal medicine, orthopaedics, rheumatology, and physiotherapy. The methods of examination developed by Cyriax have been grafted on to standard orthopaedic assessment techniques as outlined in Apley and others. The books by McRae on fracture management and clinical orthopaedic examination are referred to in most chapters. We would like to acknowledge the contribution of these authors to the field of musculo-skeletal medicine and acknowledge the use we have made of these sources in the preparation of this book.

Mr M. Clancey has given a great deal to the book through his very detailed editorial comment and we thank him for his care and patience with this project. We also thank Mr F. Morris for his comments on the manuscript.

We thank Mr Nigel Kidner for the excellent artwork and the Medical Illustration Departments of the Northern General Hospital and the Royal Hallamshire Hospital for the photographic work, as well as Dr David Moore, Consultant Radiologist, for his help in obtaining the X-rays.

We thank the British Association for Accident and Emergency Medicine for permission to use the guideline on the management of scaphoid fractures and also Miss Alison MacFarlane, Senior Physiotherapist, for the demonstration of ankle strapping.

Lastly, we would like to thank Diana, Katy, Alistair, and Veronique for their assistance and patience in putting up with us during the writing of this book!

Further reading

1. Apley, A. G. and Solomon, L. (1995). *Apley's system of orthopaedics and fractures* (7th edn). Butterworth–Heinemann, Oxford.
2. Cyriax, J. H. and Cyriax, P. J. (1993). *Cyriax's illustrated manual of orthopaedic medicine* (2nd edn). Butterworth–Heinemann, Oxford.
3. McRae, R. (1994). *Practical fracture management* (3rd edn). Churchill Livingstone, Edinburgh.

Contents

Dose schedules are being continually revised and new side effects recognized. Oxford University Press makes no representation, express or implied, that the drug dosages in this book are correct. For these reasons the reader is strongly urged to consult the pharmaceutical company's printed instructions before administering any of the drugs recommended in this book.

CHAPTER 1

Musculo-skeletal problems: introduction— the scope of musculo-skeletal medicine

Key points

- Musculo-skeletal problems are common!
- An average department will see 2000+ ankle sprains per year, but it might miss the diagnosis in the 1 case of osteomyelitis.
- This book sets out to give a clear method of assessing patients with musculo-skeletal problems.
- Take the best possible history.
- Examine the patient systematically.
- Investigate appropriately.
- Record the assessment in the notes.
- Arrange appropriate follow-up with advice on where and when to seek help if symptoms continue or get worse.

The challenge of musculo-skeletal medicine

Musculo-skeletal problems account for an estimated 3.5 million accident and emergency attendances each year.

Many sprains, bruises, and aches will be self-limiting conditions only requiring simple advice. However, there are many diagnostic dilemmas facing accident and emergency (A&E) clinicians and general practitioners (GPs) in everyday practice, for example:

- Which acutely injured knee needs specialist referral.
- Which 1 of the 1000 patients presenting with back pain requires surgery for nerve root or spinal cord compression?
- Which 1 of the 100 children presenting with a non-functioning upper limb will have osteomyelitis?
- Which of the patients presenting with foot pain will have a major vascular occlusion?
- Which of the patients presenting with an acute joint effusion will have septic arthritis?

Musculo-skeletal problems are often easily diagnosed and the treatment is straightforward. Conversely, some problems are rare but important to diagnose if life- or limb-threatening problems are to be prevented. The skill is to recognize those conditions where urgent referral and treatment are required. The magnitude of the task is indicated by reference to Table 1.1. Most patients, but not all, will have a simple ankle sprain.

Table 1.1 • Numbers of patients presenting in 1 year with ankle problems to an average A&E department (50 000 new patients per annum).

Simple ankle sprain	2200
Severe ankle sprain	260
Ankle fracture	470
Soft-tissue infection	160
Non-trauma	80
Tendon ruptures	5
Osteomyelitis	1 in 2–3 years

Adopting a close 'mind set' that all ankle problems are either sprained or fractured will inevitably lead to misdiagnosis.

The aims of this book are:

- To set out a clear *method* of history taking and examination for musculo-skeletal problems presenting to A&E departments.
- To *contrast* those conditions where there is a clear history of injury with non-traumatic musculo-skeletal problems.
- To provide a *system* that encourages the consideration of some of the rarer diagnoses.
- To *discuss* the principles of treatment and referral for patients with musculo-skeletal problems.

Fractures and the differential diagnosis in musculo-skeletal injury

The routine diagnosis and treatment of fractures is comprehensively covered in many texts (see McRae or Apley). However, there are certain fractures that must remain in the differential diagnosis of musculo-skeletal pain even when the initial radiographs are normal. Common examples of this are the scaphoid and stress fractures. There are also some fractures that are difficult radiological diagnoses. For example, failure to spot an osteochondral fracture of the talus may result in the patient being treated for a sprained ankle. Fractures that cause diagnostic difficulty are included in this book.

The role of the A&E department in the management of musculo-skeletal problems

In acute injury the role of the A&E department is clearly to assess the patient, provide the necessary immediate care, and to refer the patient appropriately. Some may question the role of A&E in the management of non-traumatic problems. However, patients will present with such conditions and they must be assessed properly or some patients with life- or limb-threatening pathology might be denied proper emergency treatment.

The follow-up of patients with injury will vary between departments. Some A&E departments will run 'soft tissue' clinics or patients can be seen in 'return clinics'. However, there is a national drive to reduce the numbers of return visits to A&E. This means that patients with moderate injury may have to be returned to the care of the general practitioner or to the orthopaedic fracture clinic.

Patients with non-traumatic problems will require similar clear referral advice. In this book there is much advice to 'refer to general practitioner'. In these cases the diagnosis may not be clear. Symptoms and signs progress over time and it is therefore necessary that patients are given clear advice to seek appropriate review.

Records and communication

Records

Due to the large number of patients presenting with musculo-skeletal injury it may be tempting to speed up the process of care by making only very brief notes. However, the duties of a doctor are clearly laid out in the Guidance from the General Medical Council:

"keep clear, accurate, and contemporaneous records which report the relevant clinical findings, the decisions made, information given to patients and any drugs or other treatment prescribed;"

This book encourages a systematic approach to history taking, examination, and treatment that can be used when recording the consultation.

Communication

This is an area of practice that often suffers as a result of pressure of work. Communication with the patient, with hospital colleagues, and with general practitioners can always be improved. Up to 50 per cent of A&E attenders will be referred for continuing care. Many departments send copies of the A&E clinical record with the patient to the ward or outpatient clinic. It is often communications with general practice that are less than ideal. When referring a patient to the care of a GP **or** informing the patient that they should see their GP if their symptoms get worse, a specific letter should be written to the patient's GP. A copy of this information should be filed in the notes. Of all letters given to patients 30 per cent may never reach the GP.

Pitfalls and how to avoid them

The wide variety of musculo-skeletal problems in accident and emergency medicine hide many pitfalls for the inexperienced, overworked, or the overconfident. Errors can be reduced by following a few guidelines:

- Obtain a good history.
- Obtain a better history.
- Obtain the best possible history.
- Follow a diagnostic routine — *check the joint above, look, feel, move, function, nerves and vessels.*
- Check the temperature and pulse in patients presenting with non-traumatic problems.

Consider sources of referred pain in non-traumatic problems:

- Obtain good quality x-rays of the injured area if indicated. Examine these x-rays methodically, asking for more experienced assistance if in doubt.
- Arrange appropriate:
  - immediate inpatient referral for patients with severe life- or limb-threatening problems;
  - immediate senior accident and emergency or orthopaedic opinion for patients with significant injuries or potentially serious problems;
  - early general practitioner review for patients with moderate disabilities or undiagnosed musculo-skeletal problems (with appropriate referral letter);
  - general advice to patients to return either to their general practitioner or to the accident department if the resolution of symptoms does not follow the expected course;
  - advice to patients who are discharged to seek further advice if their symptoms get worse or do not resolve (after 7–10 days).

Further reading

1. Apley, A. G. and Solomon, L. (1995). *Apley's system of orthopaedics and fractures* (7th edn). Butterworth–Heinemann, Oxford.
2. General Medical Council (1995). *Duties of a doctor.* General Medical Council, London.
3. McRae, R. (1994). *Practical fracture management* (3rd edn). Churchill Livingstone, Edinburgh.

CHAPTER 2

Patient assessment

Key points

- 90 per cent of patients with soft-tissue problems present after an episode of trauma. Management is often straightforward.

- 10 per cent of patients present with musculo-skeletal pain with no history of trauma. **These patients require careful assessment**.

- **If** there is no history of trauma exclude sepsis, ischaemic syndromes, referred pain, and epiphyseal problems.

Develop a system of assessment

- **History**
  - *Mechanism of injury;*
  - *Symptoms and the progress of these symptoms;*
  - *Previous injury or significant medical problems;*
- **Examine**
  - *Joint above, look, feel, move, function, nerves, and vessels.*
- **X-ray**
  - *Use guidelines and department policy but X-ray when in doubt.*
- **Follow-up**
  - *Give clear advice.*

Pitfalls

- Failure to appreciate the different spectrum of diagnoses in injured and non-injured patients;
- Adopting a closed 'mind set' (e.g. all ankles are either broken or sprained);
- Failure to admit lack of knowledge of these 'simple problems' (problems that may be highly complex). Many pitfalls are 'classic' errors well recorded in textbooks;
- Failure to take a proper history;
- Failure to examine properly using a system;
- Failure to X-ray. In spite of many guidelines a patient still feels aggrieved if they are the 1:100 that the guideline missed;
- Failure to give clear follow-up instructions;
- Failure to record all of above!

Differentiation between trauma and non-trauma

Injury accounts for 90 per cent of musculo-skeletal problems encountered in an A&E department. However, failure to consider non-traumatic causes of limb pain is a common cause for misdiagnosis and may lead to severe disability or even life-threatening problems; for example, a slipped upper femoral epiphysis, septic arthritis, or referred cardiac or abdominal pain.

In every patient with a musculo-skeletal problem consider: Is there a definite history of trauma compatible with the patient's complaints? Possible clinical situations include:

1. A clear history of injury with symptoms commencing at the time of injury. The symptoms are compatible with the mechanism of injury and are following the expected clinical course.
2. No history of trauma elicited.
3. A history of minor trauma, but no clear link to the patient's symptoms and the symptoms are more severe than expected.
4. A history of trauma, but the symptoms are not following the expected clinical course.

> **Beware patients in categories 2–3–4**
> **What are you missing?**
> **Take a detailed history**

Trauma, the spectrum of injury (Fig. 2.1)

A major problem in the assessment of acute musculo-skeletal injuries is a lack of precision in diagnosis. A 'sprain' covers a huge *spectrum of injury*, from the minor self-limiting to the permanently disabling. Only by a careful history and examination will the doctor be able to define the severity of injury. It may only be by repeated examination over a period of time that the true extent of injury is established.

Trauma, the history

Mechanism of injury, direction, magnitude and duration of force, symptoms and progress, previous history, patient's expected level of activity

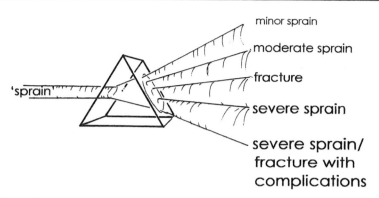

Fig. 2.1 ● Spectrum of diagnosis in acute injury.

Mechanism of injury

A clear history is the key to the accurate diagnosis in traumatic injury. An understanding of the *exact* mechanism of the injury should produce a mental picture of the *direction, magnitude,* and *duration* of forces applied to the injured part. Fig. 2.2 and Box 2.1 list some of the histories that one might see recorded in A&E notes.

The history given in **A**, Box 2.1 gives **no** idea of the mechanism of injury. It only states the *circumstances* in which the injury occurred, i.e. playing football. The injury could have been a direct blow, a fall on to the knee, a sudden onset of pain in the knee while running, or any other mechanism. Such a history is useless in the diagnosis of the problem.

Box 2.1 ● Mechanism of injury

A Injured right knee while playing football?
B Injured right knee, in a tackle, while playing football.
C Injured right knee, in a tackle during football, was taking weight on the right leg, opponent struck lateral side of the knee, knee bent inwards, and had immediate pain on the inside of the knee.

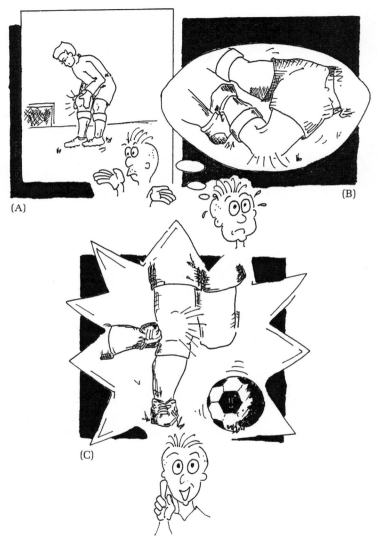

Fig. 2.2 ● Mechanism of injury; form a clear *mental image* of the magnitude, direction and duration of forces causing the injury (for explanation see text).

The history as recorded in **B** is more specific regarding the circumstances of the injury, but again there is little information regarding the true *mechanism* of injury.

Part **C** gives a very good description of the mechanism of injury. Such a description allows a *mental visualization* of the injury with many clear clues as to the possible diagnosis. This mental picture of the injury process is a key to the diagnosis.

Symptoms and progress

The patient is asked to describe their symptoms and if these symptoms have progressed over time since the accident. For example, a sudden and complete loss of function ('getting carried off') increases the index of suspicion of a more severe injury.

The main symptoms of musculo-skeletal injury are pain, swelling, and loss of function. Also ask about other symptoms such as paraesthesia and other injuries.

Past history and previous injuries

Most injuries are acute, but some are an acute episode in a more chronic pattern. The investigation and treatment of an 'acute on chronic' injury may be slightly different. The management of a recent, simple inversion of the ankle may be different from repeated inversion injuries. Ask the patient if they have any other significant medical conditions or are taking any medication.

Level of activity

Patient expectations are an important consideration in the management of musculo-skeletal injuries. It could be argued that all injuries should receive the same treatment, but with limited resources this would be impossible. For example, an office clerk with no strenuous leisure pastimes suffering an inversion injury of the ankle with 80 per cent of function will probably notice no interference with their lifestyle. Conversely, a steeplejack or professional athlete demand as near 100 per cent function as is possible. Appreciation of these individual expectations represents good patient management.

Trauma, examination

Joint above, look, feel, move, function, nerves, vascular supply

1. Begin the examination by having the patient in a relaxed position. Start by examining the joint proximal to the injury (or spine if indicated) ('Joint above').
2. Follow standard orthopaedic practice, using the *look, feel, move, function* method.
3. Complete the examination by checking circulation to the limbs and testing neural function distal to the injury.

Joint above

It is always good practice to check the joint proximal to the injury. Usually there is no injury, and by commencing the examination in this fashion you will make contact with the patient, not cause pain, and gain confidence and rapport with the patient. Occasionally, there will be positive findings and an injury will be diagnosed that would otherwise have been missed.

Look

Close observation of the patient will provide many clues to the diagnosis. The patient may walk abnormally, may hold the affected limb in a certain way, and a general examination of the patient's appearance may indicate the severity of the pain.

Compare the affected limb or area to the unaffected side. Although gross areas of swelling and bruising may be obvious, subtle areas of swelling or deformity will be missed unless a direct comparison is made. Before proceeding to examine the affected part, this is an appropriate stage to examine the proximal part of the limb, especially if there is a possibility that the pain may be due to radiation from the neck, back, and proximal joints.

Feel

This examination should proceed in a logical and practised fashion. Each joint will have key points where tenderness is sought following specific injuries. These areas are referred to under 'Specific joint examination' in subsequent chapters.

Commence palpation at a point distant from the area of injury. For example, palpate the fibular head in an ankle injury to exclude damage to that structure and to gain the patient's confidence. The rest of the examination should be systematic, palpating with a single finger those areas where associated injuries *might* be found. For example, in ankle injury palpate the tibia down to the medial malleolus, medial ligament, the metatarsal joint, especially the base of the 5th metatarsal and the tendo-Achilles. With practice, this takes less than 30 seconds and a wealth of information is obtained. Once these are have been examined, then the lateral malleolus and lateral ligament complex can be examined in detail.

At this stage, the presence of crepitus may also be felt (do not try to elicit crepitus as it is very painful). The presence of swelling around the joint should lead the examiner to test for the presence or absence of an effusion within the joint, for example the knee joint (see Chapter 11).

Move (Figs 2.3 A–D)

- active range ⎫
- passive range ⎭ Joint function
- resisted movement — muscles/tendon
- stress testing — ligaments.

The 'look' and 'feel' parts of the examination will help to isolate the injured *area*. It is movement that gives clues to the exact *structure* involved.

If the muscle, tendon, or muscular insertion is damaged then characteristically there will be pain on resisted movement.

If a ligament is damaged then there may be pain on stressing the ligament or abnormal movement over the joint.

Definitions:
Capsular pattern — A characteristic limitation in movement of a joint when there is a joint effusion or inflammation of the capsule, e.g. capsular pattern of the shoulder joint (for example, traumatic effusion or adhesive capsulitis) there is limitation in abduction, external rotation in the neutral position, and internal rotation in extension (arm up behind back).

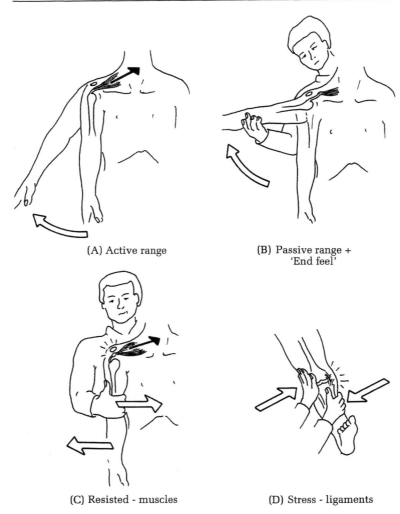

(A) Active range

(B) Passive range +
'End feel'

(C) Resisted - muscles

(D) Stress - ligaments

Fig. 2.3 • Move: four basic types of movement to examine. (A) **Active range**. Patient moves the limb, muscles and ligaments are being stretched, joint is in motion. (B) **Passive range**. The examiner moves the joint, ligaments are stretched, the joint is moving. Muscles are not acting but will be stretched at the limits of range. (C) **Resisted movement**. Muscles and tendons active. The joint is not moving, ligaments are not being stretched. (D) **Stress testing**. Examiner looks for abnormal mobility of ligaments.

End feel — End (of range of movement) feel. This is the sensation felt at the end of range of movement, usually shortened to 'end feel'. It may be described as 'empty' when there is a feeling that there is no resistance to continued movement, e.g. when stressing a ruptured ligament or 'hard' or 'solid' when the ligament is intact.

Active range

Joint injuries commonly produce characteristic limitations of movement, e.g. an acute effusion within the shoulder joint will limit external rotation and abduction, whereas flexion, extension, and internal rotation in neutral are relatively pain-free. Such a characteristic pattern or limited movement is called the 'Capsular pattern' for that joint.

Passive range

Movements performed by the examiner may also reveal the typical limitation of movement of the capsular pattern. If there is pain-free movement of the joint, over a limited range, then this makes acute inflammation within the joint much less likely.

In testing the passive range of movement of a joint, the examiner should gauge the *end feel* of that movement. For example, when examining the knee joint, if there is a block to full extension, the experienced examiner can sometimes differentiate between a mechanical block, for instance due to a loose body, or by the capsular limitation or capsular pattern of limitation of movement caused by an effusion (Fig. 2.4).

Passive movement will stretch muscle groups at the extremes of joint movement so pain in this instance may be due to muscle injury or muscle problems (Figs 2.5, 2.6).

Resisted movement

In testing resisted movement, the joints do not move, but the patient presses against the examiner's hand to test specific muscle groups. Pain on such movement indicates that the *musculotendon* unit is the site of the problem. This may be confirmed by pain on passive stretch of the muscle. For example, if when testing resisted eversion of the ankle joint,

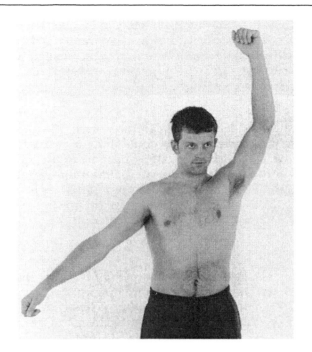

(A)

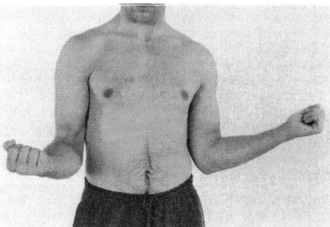

(B)

Fig. 2.4 • Capsular pattern of restriction in joint movement. When a joint is inflamed there is a characteristic limitation in movement. For the shoulder joint, this is limitation in external rotation and in abduction.

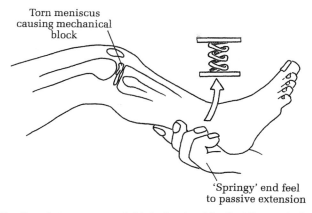

Fig. 2.5 • Passive movement. Note the 'end feel' at the end of passive range. This may be; 'springy' or 'rubbery' in a mechanical block as with a torn meniscus or loose body. 'Inhibited' by muscle spasm. 'Empty' if normal restricting structures lost.

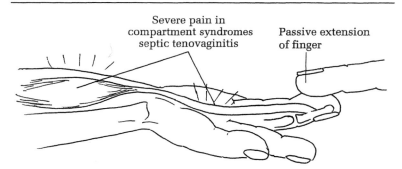

Fig. 2.6 • Passive movement will stretch muscle groups at the extremes of their movement, for example, in compartment syndrome or a septic tenovaginitis.

the patient indicates that they feel pain at the base of the 5th metatarsal, then the diagnosis is probably an avulsion fracture of the insertion of the peroneus brevis (Fig. 2.7).

Resisted movement also helps to assess the *integrity* of musculotendon units, a striking example of this is straight-leg

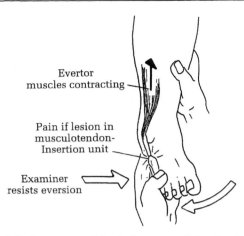

Evertor
muscles contracting

Pain if lesion in
musculotendon-
Insertion unit

Examiner
resists eversion

Fig. 2.7 ● Resisted movement tests the musculotendon-insertion unit. Ankle eversion against resistance causes pain in a fracture of the base of 5th metatarsal, the insertion of peroneus brevis tendon.

raising in a knee injury which confirms the presence and continuity of the quadriceps tendon, the patellar insertion, and the patellar tendon. (In this case the resisted movement is against gravity.)

Stress testing

Stress testing abnormal movement indicates that the normal factors maintaining stability have been significantly damaged.

WARNING! — *Muscle power* is one of the major factors influencing joint stability. In the injured patient, reflex muscle spasm may prevent the demonstration of ligamentous instability. If instability is to be demonstrated, then the patient must be as relaxed as possible and have some confidence in the examiner. Distracting the patient by chatting to the them while performing the test aids diagnostic accuracy.

Commonly used stress tests are the anterior draw test (ankle), anterior draw test and collateral ligament testing (knee), and testing for the collateral ligaments of the fingers, especially metacarpphalangeal joint of the thumb.

In the acutely injured patient, it is quite possible that a ligament may be completely ruptured and yet intense protective muscle spasm may make it impossible to demonstrate abnormal movement of the joint.

Function

Observe the patient using the injured limb for normal function. In lower limb injuries, try to get the patient to walk, crouch, and kneel (this may have to be after X-ray if there is a strong suspicion of fracture). Omission of this part of the examination can lead to significant errors, for example in the examination of a child who is not weight-bearing it is quite common to find absolutely no abnormalities on examination with the child lying on a couch. However, when the child does try to walk, it is quite obvious that there is something significantly wrong by their abnormal gait or their absolute refusal to bear weight.

Nerves and vascular supply

This must be a routine part of the examination of all musculo-skeletal problems.

Trauma, investigation

Plain X-ray

Patient with definite history of injury

In most A&E departments, the commonest investigation is that of plain radiography to exclude a bony injury. While there are some signs of soft-tissue injury to be found on X-ray, these are not common.

A normal X-ray does not necessarily exclude a fracture. Common examples of this are the scaphoid and stress fractures. Fractures may also be missed due to the failure to X-ray the proper part (e.g. hand instead of finger) or due to inadequate X-rays, more common in large central joints or spine.

Correct interpretation of the X-ray is central to patient management. Failure to diagnose a fracture may lead to inappropriate advice or inappropriate treatment. Develop a system of X-ray interpretation to minimize the risks of error.

A system of interpretation is as follows:

1. Take a case history and examine the patient.
2. Identify that the X-rays belong to the correct patient and show the correct side.
3. Examine the X-rays for quality and ensure that the injured parts have been adequately demonstrated and the films are of suitable exposure. There should always be films in two planes, preferably taken at right angles, to each other.
4. Examine A, B, C, S, **A**lignment, **B**ones, **C**artilage, **S**oft tissues (from Nicholson and Driscoll).

Further assistance can be obtained by experienced radiographers reporting films. Every A&E department should have a reporting system where X-rays are seen by experienced radiologists, any errors in interpretation are recognized and appropriate follow-up action taken.

Stress X-rays

The presence of pain limits the usefulness of stress X-rays in A&E departments. There are some injuries, such as the rupture of the ulnar collateral ligament of the metacarpophalangeal joint of the thumb, where the installation of local anaesthetic into the painful area may allow stress X-rays to be performed. Examples of such procedures are given under the specific subject areas.

Diagnostic ultrasound

Ultrasound is becoming increasingly available and of increasing use in the diagnosis of musculo-skeletal problems. Swelling cysts, tendons and paratendonous structures, and the presence of joint effusion can all be studied by the use of ultrasound.

Other investigations

The further diagnosis of musculo-skeletal problems may lie outside the scope of the A&E department, and these could include:

- *Examination under anaesthesia* this allows proper examination of the joints and formal stress testing.
- *Magnetic resonance imaging* (MRI) is fast becoming the 'gold standard' of imaging in musculo-skeletal problems. The main bars to its use are availability and cost. In future it is likely that this investigation will become much more widely used in the diagnosis of musculo-skeletal injuries and soft-tissue problems.
- *Computed tomography* (CT) is of some use in the diagnosis of musculo-skeletal problems. Images difficult to obtain by plain X-rays (e.g. the cervicothoracic junction, small bones in the foot, or fine detail of the wrist) may be easier to visualize by using CT scanning. This technique will be more widely used in the future for difficult diagnostic problems.
- *Arthroscopy* of the knee is well established as both a diagnostic and therapeutic procedure. Modern arthroscopes now make it possible to perform arthroscopy on a much wider range of joints such as wrist, ankle, and even the hip and shoulder. Again, these techniques will become more widely used for difficult problems but are outside the scope of most A&E departments.

Non-trauma, assessment

History

Assessment of these patients takes time

Differentiation from acute trauma

Patients may present with a musculo-skeletal problem but with no history of injury. Alternatively, the patient may say that they have hurt themselves, but it is only on closer questioning that it becomes clear that there has been no *specific* episode of injury. In such cases, think of the diagnoses of sepsis, ischaemia, or referred pain (Box 2.2) or those listed in 'Softer tissues' (Chapter 4). Failure to *consider* such problems may lead to these important conditions being missed.

Box 2.2 ● No specific episode of injury

S Exclude sepsis

I Exclude ischaemia

R Exclude referred pain from chest/abdomen/spine

Onset and progress — The most common symptom is pain. The patient should be asked, in detail, about the onset of pain. Was it gradual? Was it sudden? Were there associated symptoms? Many serious pathologies may cause severe pain with very few findings on examination.

Of special significance is the presence of pain at night that keeps the patient awake. This usually indicates a severe inflammatory process and such pain should always be taken seriously.

Severe pain at night = severe pathology

Type of pain — Is the pain throbbing in nature, toothache-like, or sharp and associated with certain movements? Ask if the pain radiates either proximally or distally in the limb. This may be an indication that the problem lies more centrally.

The presence of aggravating or relieving factors — Ask if the patient has participated in any unusual activity in the period leading up to the onset of symptoms, or has recently significantly increased the level of an activity (e.g. doubling the running distance) which would be unusual for that patient. Other aggravating or relieving factors are noted.

Previous history — Note previous medical history, especially if there have been similar problems in the past. Exclude problems with other joints or a history of arthritis. Exclude many of the more common diseases such as diabetes.

Associated symptoms — Ask if there are any other symptoms such as back problems, eye problems, inflammatory bowel symptoms, genitourinary symptoms, recent illnesses, and respiratory-tract infection.

Examination — no history of trauma

While the principles of examination are identical to those listed above, there are some important differences.

General examination

Attention should be paid to the general state of the patient. Are they pale, tired, drawn; indicating a significant lack of sleep. Do they have any stigmata of systemic disease or of systemic arthritis? Are there any skin rashes?

It is good practice to measure the vital signs. The temperature and pulse rate should be recorded.

Sites of possible pathology should always be checked in a systemic and thorough fashion. The spine should be examined as should proximal joints.

Examine the chest/abdomen/spine

Joint above — In non-traumatic problems always examine more proximally. The limb as a whole needs to be examined, and often the spine. Pain radiating from a central focus does not always follow dermatomal or peripheral nerve distribution.

Look — Always compare limbs where there is no specific history of injury. The signs of swelling or deformity may be very subtle and very easily missed.

Feel — Check if there is any difference in temperature as well as careful palpation for points of tenderness.

Move — The use of active range, passive range, and resisted movement all help to identify the structures involved. For example, in a patient presenting with pain around the elbow joint, if it is found that there is full range of movement of the elbow joint but that there is pain on resisted extension of the wrist, along with pain on passive flexion of the wrist, then the diagnosis is almost certainly lateral epicondylitis (tennis elbow). **Function** — The signs on examination may be minimal, but when the patient is asked to use the limb normally the lack of function may then be obvious.

Nerves and vessels — Ischaemia, compartment syndrome, neural compression, and referred pain include some of the most serious causes of non-traumatic soft-tissue problems. Failure to examine the pulses and to perform a neurological assessment will lead to errors in diagnosis.

Investigation — no history of injury

The nature of investigations in such a patient will depend on the presentation and clinical signs. For example, if there is an acutely swollen joint, then investigations should include:

- Aspiration of the joint (depending on local protocol). Fluid is sent for microscopy looking for cells and bacteria, polarizing light microscopy for crystals, and culture and sensitivity of microorganisms;
- Full blood count and ESR;
- Uric, calcium, and phosphate levels;
- Rheumatoid factor.

In addition, X-rays of the painful area may well be required, although many serious conditions may have a normal X-ray.

Pitfalls and how to avoid them

Communication problems, children, non-traumatic soft-tissue problems, more than one injury, documentation, further communication.

Failure to take an adequate history (communication problems)

This is the most frequent and often the most serious error made in A&E practice. This may be due to:

- Lack of time to take an adequate history;
- Problems with communication in patients where English is not their first language;
- Children;
- Other communication problems such as deafness, learning disorders, and dementia.

Without an adequate history it may be impossible to make an accurate diagnosis.

Children's musculo-skeletal problems

Musculo-skeletal problems in children require special mention. Often the pain is not well localized. Even in the presence of significant injuries such as a spiral fracture of tibia, there may be absolutely nothing to find on examination, specifically there may be no swelling, no bruising, and no localized tenderness. A child not using a limb requires a very careful evaluation, and consideration should be given to X-raying the whole of the affected limb. If no obvious cause for the child's pain is found, then it is wise to seek a further opinion or to bring this child back for review within 1–3 days.

Non-traumatic musculo-skeletal problems

The range of possible diagnoses in patients with no history of trauma is extensive. Because of the rarity of some of these problems, it is understandable how such diagnoses might not be considered in the management of such patients. Inexperienced A&E staff, therefore, must be aware of the potential for serious problems in patients with musculo-skeletal pain but with no history of injury.

Multiple injuries

The commonest presentation is of a single injury to a specific part of the body. Problems arise due to a number of injuries being present in the same patient. There is an inevitable tendency to skimp on the history and examination of each of these specific injuries to concentrate on the injury which appears to be worse at the time. Examine and document all injuries fully and treat each injury carefully.

Failure of documentation

This is a recurring theme in cases where there is complaint or litigation. Often the staff involved will have followed good management practice but their recording of findings may be woefully inadequate. This makes it very difficult to defend any such actions. Failure of documentation may, in part, be due to inexperience and uncertainty regarding terminology, and notation regarding range of movements of joint. These issues will be clearly explained later in sections on the individual body areas. Significant negative findings, as well as positive findings, should be recorded. In medical legal matters it is assumed 'if it has not been recorded, it has not been done'.

Failure of communication

There is an increasing demand for improvements to be made in communication, especially between the A&E departments and general practice. If you are referring a patient to their general practitioner for follow-up then it is good practice to write a letter stating the problem.

Further reading

1. Apley, A. G. and Solomon, L. (1995). *Apley's system of orthopaedics and fractures* (7th edn). Butterworth–Heinemann, Oxford.
2. Corrigan, B. and Maitland, G. D. (1994). *Musculo-skeletal and sports injuries.* Butterworth–Heinemann, Oxford
3. Cyriax, J. (1982). *Textbook of orthopaedic medicine.* Vol. 1 Diagnosis on soft tissue lesions. Baillière Tindall, London.
4. Cyriax, J. H. and Cyriax, P. J. (1993). *Cyriax's illustrated manual of orthopaedic medicine* (2nd edn). Butterworth–Heinemann, Oxford.
5. McRae, R. (1990). *Clinical orthopaedic examination* (3rd edn). Churchill Livingstone, Edinburgh.
6. Nicholson, D. A. and Driscoll, P. A. (1995). *ABC of emergency radiology.* BMJ Publications, London.

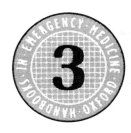

CHAPTER 3

Soft-tissue injury and repair: relevance to treatment

Key points

- The process of repair after injury is described in three stages:
  1. The inflammatory phase (days 0–3): causes pain, swelling inhibition of function — treat to reduce inflammation, swelling, and pain.
  2. The proliferative phase (days 3–7): results in laying down weak collagen — treat by protected careful activity.
  3. The maturation phase (7–28+ days) results in maturation of collagen and remodelling — treat by graded return to full function.
- Muscle injury may be caused by a direct blow or forceful contractions tearing the muscle. Repair is often slow and can leave permanent scars. *Compartment syndrome* and *myositis ossificans* are serious sequelae to muscle injury.
- Tendon injury may be overlooked (e.g. Achilles tendon). Total ruptures are often treated surgically.
- Ligament injury presents a *spectrum* of damage from minor self-limiting partial tears to complete ruptures of ligament complexes.
- Closed nerve injury is often treated conservatively (apart from pressure on the spinal cord or nerve roots which may be a surgical emergency).

Soft-tissue healing

An injury to the soft tissues, results in a complex healing process. This will lead to the restoration of normal tissue or the production of scar tissue. The minor differences that occur in the healing of each separate soft tissue will not be discussed in detail. Essentially, the overall process is the same whether discussing the healing of muscle, tendon, or ligament.

Wound healing

Wound healing is classically divided into three phases.

Inflammatory phase (0–3 days)

At the time of injury, blood vessels in the area are damaged and mediators of acute inflammation are released causing initial vasoconstriction, closely followed by dilation. As blood flow in the area increases, the permeability of the vessels also increases. Platelets bind to exposed collagen. Fibronectin and fibrin provide crosslinks to the collagen producing a temporary plug to prevent further haemorrhage. Phospholipids are released by the collagen which also stimulates the clotting mechanism. Polymorphonuclear leucocytes and monocytes act as macrophages to remove necrotic tissue.

The chemical mediators also increase the sensitivity of pain receptors, causing increased pain perception in and around the injured area. All the clinical symptoms and signs observed immediately after an acute injury can therefore be accounted for by the process of acute inflammation. Reduction in the severity of the inflammatory phase is the first step in the treatment and rehabilitation of a soft-tissue injury. If the inflammatory phase is prolonged then the continuation of pain leads to neurological reflex muscle inhibition that will result in loss of function and prolonged rehabilitation.

Towards the end of the inflammatory phase there is a migration of fibroblasts into the area that will produce the collagen necessary for the next phase.

Proliferative phase (3–7 days)

The duration of this phase is from the third day up to a week post-injury. Fibroblasts, myofibroblasts, and endothelial cells are encouraged to proliferate by growth factors produced by the platelets and macrophages. This forms a new capillary system, the fibroblasts produce a developing extracellular matrix, i.e. the basis of granulation tissue. However, this stage of transition results in the tensile strength of the tissue being at its lowest level. Unnecessary stress at this time must be avoided. This has to be emphasized to the individual as the temptation to return to work or sport may set back the repair process.

The undifferentiated cells may form abnormal types of connective tissue with mucoid, hyaline, myxoid degeneration, calcification or bony metaplasia occurring.

The collagen being formed is Type II, thin and weak. As the scar matures it develops pain and pressure-sensitive nerve endings. The new capillary system is also weak and may tear easily. There is increased fluid in the area due to extensive vascularity. This also produces tenderness in the area.

After 1 week, the tensile strength improves and the Type II collagen will shortly be replaced by stronger Type I collagen. At this time contraction of the wound may also occur, reducing its size.

Maturation phase (7 days up to many months)

Stress applied to the maturing collagen during this phase results in increased strength of the wound due to the improved organization of the fibres. This phase may last for months with the structure undergoing continuous remodelling. Vascularity decreases leading to a whiter and less-sensitive tissue.

Relevance to treatment principles

The treatment of soft-tissue injury is a *dynamic process* that aims to follow the patterns of normal repair:

• Initially (days 0–3), to reduce the acute inflammatory response;

- Then, to commence gentle return to function, often with the use of strapping or support as the repair process is incomplete and the joints may still be weak, (3–14 days);
- Finally (7 days to months), to commence a programme of gradual return to full function.

There is no definite time-scale for each of the treatment phases, just as there is no set time-scale to the physiological healing process. Each injury will take a variable time to heal; **beware** those patients who are taking longer than expected or whose symptoms are more severe than expected. Is the diagnosis correct or have they developed a complication? Similarly, **beware** the keen athlete who wishes to resume maximum function 2 days after a significant soft-tissue injury. They should be carefully assessed and advised that a too-early return to competitive sport may not be in the best interests of their own natural healing process.

Treatment during the inflammatory phase

The main objectives are to reduce swelling and inflammation. **R**est, **I**ce, **C**ompression, and **E**levation (**RICE**) is the simple advice given to patients. This must be explained fully, warning the patient about possible adverse effects:

— give details for the proper application of ice to prevent skin burns (a towel or flannel is placed over the injured part and crushed ice or a bag of frozen peas applied for 10 minutes);

— the proper use of support, the problems of bandages that may become too tight due to swelling;

— elevation must be with the injured limb above the heart (e.g. lying down with the leg elevated to 30–45 degrees or the arm resting on a pillow on the arm of a chair (Fig. 3.1).

Drug treatment

Analgesia is advised. Paracetamol is safe and effective for most minor to moderate soft-tissue injuries. There is some weak evidence that non-steroidal anti-inflammatory agents may reduce swelling more effectively, but these benefits must

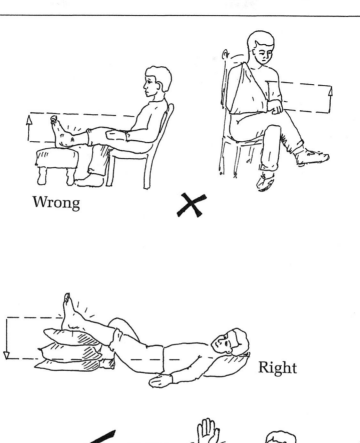

Wrong

Right

Fig. 3.1 ● Proper limb elevation. Give clear instructions to the patient regarding proper elevation above the heart.

be weighed against their problems, especially in the elderly, those with peptic ulcer disease, and asthmatics (see Chapter 5).

Topical non-steroidal formulations such as dressings and gels have theoretical attractions, but there is little hard evidence to support their use routinely in soft-tissue injury.

Treatment during the proliferative phase

A phase of protected function should be encouraged as soon as pain allows, for example the patient with a moderate ankle sprain who cannot bear weight may require crutches, but they are advised to try to get their foot to the ground as soon as the pain allows. Supports and bandages may be very effective during this phase. However, proper support and strapping is a skilled and a time-consuming process. Many 'routine' strappings used in A&E work do not give effective support (for example, see Stirrup strapping for ankle sprain).

Treatment during the maturation phase

> **The rehabilitation phase is probably the most important phase in the recovery from a soft-tissue injury.**

The patient is advised to gradually return to their normal activity. They should' 'walk before they can run', gently kick a light ball before they try a proper match ball, and then they might be ready to have a light practice session. The aim of this advice is to try and regain the strength and stability of the joint, which is highly dependent on normal muscle power and neural reflexes.

Muscles: anatomy and physiology

Each muscle has an *origin* where it is attached to the bone (usually). The fleshy part of the muscle may originate directly on to the periosteum (quadriceps to femur) or there may be a tendon linking the muscle belly to the origin (e.g. the long and short heads of biceps brachii).

The muscle belly consists of striated skeletal muscle fibres. These may travel the whole length of the muscle. Each fibre is surrounded by a membrane, the sarcolemma. The outer coating of the sarcolemma fuses with the tendon fibres. The tendon connects the muscle to its *insertion* where the fibrous tissue of the tendon blends with the periosteum of the bone.

Muscle contraction

Muscles produce movement, give shock absorption, and act as energy-storing devices (this action being more evident in tendons). Each muscle fibre contains several hundred myofibrils. Each myofibril has about 1500 myosin filaments and 3000 actin filaments that interdigitate to cause contraction. The sarcoplasm surrounding the filaments provides the nutrients, salts, and energy required for contraction.

Sarcoplasmic reticulum surrounds the myofibrils. The greater the density of this structure the faster the potential contraction of the muscle.

Types of muscle

I   Red. Slow twitch. Aerobic. Plentiful mitochondria. Postural muscles (erector spinae).

II   White. Fast twitch. Anaerobic. Glycolysis for energy. Fatigue quickly.

IIA   High oxidative.

IIB   Low oxidative.

Muscles: injury and treatment

Injury

Intrinsic injuries occur due to excessive tension.

A *minor muscular tear* involves minimal fibre disruption and may be termed as a pull or strain. It may present as muscle soreness lasting a few days.

A *partial tear* will show an extramuscular haematoma plus bruising, or an intramuscular haematoma with general tender swelling.

A major muscular tear incorporates tearing and bleeding. A complete tear involves loss of function, although other muscles or other parts of the muscle may continue to allow reasonable function (e.g. the short head of biceps rupture). **Extrinsic injuries** consist of a direct contusion.

Aggravating factors

1. Lack of fitness;
2. Lack of attention to self-care and management/injury avoidance by complying with regular stretching and warm-up routines;
3. Previous injury and tethering scar tissue;
4. Previous immobilization will have produced a deficient contractile unit.

Complications

Compartment syndrome may complicate any muscle injury. Severe unremitting pain made worse by passive stretch of the muscle is the cardinal pointer to this diagnosis (see p. 000.)

Myositis ossificans may develop due bony metaplasia of undifferentiated mesenchymal cells. This is a major complication of this type of injury. It most commonly occurs after the aggressive rehabilitation of a contusion injury. Stretching and other active physiotherapy should be delayed in such patients. For example, with quadriceps haematoma if the knee cannot be flexed past 90 degrees then rest, ice, ultrasound, and crutches are used until the acute phase has settled.

Treatment

Injury to a muscle belly is almost always treated by conservative measures. Minor muscle pulls and strains require a period of rest, ice, and analgesia followed by a period of gradually increasing activity. Advice is given on the importance of proper stretching and general fitness.

More severe tears will require a period of strict rest and then a period of supervised rehabilitation.

Complete ruptures of a muscle *belly* are difficult to repair (tendons can be repaired).

Direct blows causing significant intramuscular haematoma will require strict rest. Ultrasound may speed resolution of the clot. If the condition is not improving as expected then suspect myositis ossificans.

Tendons: anatomy and physiology

Tendons are cords of highly organized bundles of Type I collagen. The cellular matrix is sparse consisting of fibrocytes. The bundles of collagen are covered in thin looser-weave fibrous tissue, the *endotenon*. The blood supply to the tendon runs in this covering. The whole tendon is sheathed in a thin layer of *epitenon*. This epitenon is continuous with the *epimysium* covering the muscle (Fig. 3.2).

The blood supply enters the tendon at its attachments, especially to muscle, and through the loose areolar tissue, the *mesotenon* that runs through the length of the tendon. The musculotendinous junction is a highly specialized structure

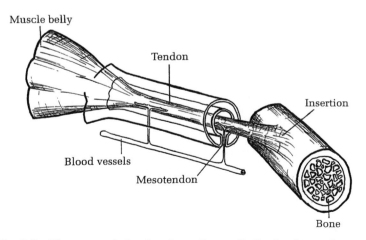

Muscle belly

Tendon

Insertion

Blood vessels

Mesotendon

Bone

Fig. 3.2 • **The musculotendon-insertion unit, the basic engine and energy transmission system of the body**. Note the blood supply to the tendon through the mesotenon. Each part of this unit is susceptible to injury.

where the bundles of collagen interdigitate with the muscle fibres and are 'welded' to the muscle cells. The *paratenon* are the loose tissues surrounding the tendon. Where the tendon changes direction or crosses a joint then the paratenon becomes thickened into a *tendon sheath*, or a *bursa* develops. These structures are lined with synovial cells and synovial fluid. They reduce the friction of the tendon at these sites of extrinsic compression. *Sesamoid bones* (e.g. patella, foot sesamoids) may develop in tendons at sites of maximum friction to reduce the wear and tear on the tendon itself. Insertions into bone are specialized areas and different types of insertion are described.

Tendons are extremely strong and can withstand strains of up to 10 kg (100 newtons) per mm^2 of tendon. For example, the flexor pollicis longus muscle has a cross-sectional area of 11 mm^2 and thus can withstand forces of over 1000 newtons.

Tendons are not rigid structures, but they stretch and recoil in response to strains placed on the structure. Under moderate stress (12 newtons per mm^2) average tendons will stretch about 2 per cent of their length.

Tendons: injury and treatment

Normal tendon can withstand great stress, and even if 75 per cent has been divided it will not break under normal loading. Tendons may be damaged by a number of mechanisms.

- They may be cut in a open wound or crushed and divided by blunt violence (e.g. the middle slip of the finger extensor tendon).
- A sudden increase in force of contraction may tear the tendon (e.g. patellar tendon rupture or closed flexor digitorum rupture).
- Spontaneous rupture may occur without a significant mechanism of injury and this can be a pitfall in diagnosis. This is probably due to degenerative disease or vascular insufficiency (e.g. Achilles or supraspinatus tendons.)

Tendon healing follows that of other collagen-rich tissues with acute inflammation, followed by laying down of granulation tissue, and then connective-tissue repair. The end result of tendon damage is likely to be a tendon that is weaker and, at worst, the site of chronic inflammatory changes (including myxoid degeneration) that interfere with function and make further damage and rupture more likely.

Treatment

Ruptured tendons generally need repair, refer to the orthopaedic team for assessment.

Partial ruptures do occur, but beware of this diagnosis as other agonist muscles may be mimicking the tendon function (e.g. in a complete rupture of the Achilles tendon foot plantar flexion is still possible due to the action of flexor hallicus longus and the long toe flexors). Seek further advice before diagnosing a partial tendon rupture.

Tendonitis true inflammation of the tendon substance is a common result of degenerative change. Minor trauma may result in aberrant repair processes which result in cystic (myxomatous) changes or even with heterotopic calcification. Treatment is difficult and often prolonged. Physiotherapy may help. Steriod injection is probably outside the treatment protocols of most A&E departments (apart from acute calcific tendinitis (p. 83)).

True tenosynovitis is rare. *Septic tenosynovitis* is a surgical emergency which needs prompt diagnosis and referral. Penetrating injuries to the hands (e.g. cat bite) are the commonest source. There is tenderness and swelling along the tendon sheath and severe pain on passive stretch of the muscle.

Stenosing tenovaginitis is a fairly common problem (e.g. trigger thumb (p. 170) and De Quervain's (p. 141)). There is thickening of the tendon sheath with local pain, a tender swelling, and clicking or locking of the tendon.

Paratendinitis crepitans (forearm, ankle) is a common overuse injury. There is generally a history of overuse and characteristic findings of swelling and crepitation. Rest is usually curative.

Ligaments: anatomy and physiology

Ligaments may be intra-articular (e.g. knee cruciate ligaments), capsular (thickenings of the joint capsule, e.g. the ankle ligaments), or extra-articular (e.g. the coracoclavicular ligaments).

They attach to bone directly or indirectly through the periosteum.

Ligaments and joint capsules consist of densely packed bundles of type I collagen and up to 10 per cent of Type III collagen. Elastin content varies from 5 per cent up to 75 per cent (ligamentum flavum).

Fibroblasts make and maintain the ligament substance. Younger ligaments have a higher number of cells and the activity of the cells appears to decrease with age. The blood supply of ligaments is via the surrounding loose fibrous tissue or by the periosteal attachments. In dense fibrous tissue, cells may be some distance from the nearest vessel, they depend on diffusion for their nutrition.

Ligaments and tendons have a vital sensory function

While ligaments have a mechanical effect on joint stability this is probably less important than the part they play as the sensory arm in the reflex muscle contractions, the major factor in joint stability. Loss of this proprioceptive function is one of the leading causes of joint instability after ligament injury. For example, a complete rupture of the anterior cruciate ligament of the knee may not be functionally important as long as there is good muscle function.

Ligaments: injury and treatment

Ligaments will tear when a deforming force exceeds the tensile strength of the structure. When a force is applied to a joint, the joint capsule, or a ligament the structure is stretched and protective muscle reflexes activated. For example, when going over on an ankle the peroneal muscles will forcibly contract to correct the inversion and the weight will shift on to the other leg. If the force is so great or if so suddenly applied that no protective reflex is possible then the ligament will take the full effect of the force and it will tear.

Ligament healing follows the same process as for other fibrous tissues. The fibrous repair will not have the same strength as the uninjured ligament and the healing process may result in lengthening of the ligament, thus allowing more joint movement. Damage to the nerve endings will result in poorer proprioceptive function. The proprioceptor-muscle reflex unit is probably more important in rehabilitation from injury than the healing of the ligament.

Ligament damage includes a whole *spectrum* of injury, from a tear of a few fibres of part of a ligament up to complete ruptures of a whole ligament complex including damage to other structures (e.g. O'Donoghue's triad in knee injury.

Injury classification

There is a system that describes ligament injuries as Grades 1, 2, and 3. In the acute situation it may be difficult to diagnose the exact grade of injury as this may require experience, time, and often special investigations.

Grade 1 — Minor sprains, partial tear of part of the ligament;
Grade 2 — Moderate sprains, complete tear of part of the ligament;
Grade 3 — Severe sprains, complete tear of all the ligament.

Common sense should allow the average practitioner to predict the severity of the injury from:

• The history, severe force = more severe injury;
• Complete loss of function = more severe injury;
• Massive swelling and loss of movement = more severe injury;
• Positive stress testing indicating a rupture (in the acute situation, protective muscle spasm makes such testing very unreliable).

Treatment

Minor sprains: Grade 1

Characterized by minor/moderate mechanism of injury, some but not total disability, moderate, localized swelling and tenderness.

This is the most common injury and the aims of treatment are:

- initial pain relief
- prevention of swelling
- early mobilization
- rehabilitation.

The methods used to treat minor sprains will vary according to local policy. Some individuals with high-functional demands may require more intensive treatment such as early physiotherapy even with a minor sprain (see Assessment). There are various methods used to recall the elements of this treatment, but we favour **RICE-R**.

R — *rest*, initially to help pain and overcome swelling;

I — application of *ice* for 10 minutes, 3 to 4 times per day (over a cloth to prevent cold burns);

C — the use of *compression* to avoid swelling;

E — *elevation* with the leg/arm above the heart to allow a true reduction in swelling;

R — *Rehabilitation*, as soon as possible (after 2–3 days) to allow early restoration of function, retraining of proprioception, and to prevent loss of muscle power.

The patient can carry out all of these activities themselves, but if they need high-functional demands in their job or leisure activities, physiotherapy may be indicated. Follow-up (if needed) is by the GP unless there is doubt over the severity of the injury or the patient requires specialist attention.

Moderate sprains: Grade 2

Characterized by significant mechanism of injury, marked swelling, unable to bear weight.

The treatment principles are the same as for minor sprains, but often crutches are required and the patient will need to be reviewed in the A&E department or fracture clinic. Physiotherapy may be indicated for the patient with high-functional demands or who requires an early return to work or sport.

Severe sprains: Grade 3

Characterized by significant mechanism of injury, massive swelling, unable to bear weight, signs of instability.

Treatment of these injuries is controversial. Logically, a completely torn ligament should require surgical repair and some do advocate this type of treatment. However, good results are also claimed for active non-surgical treatment. This regime consists of functional bracing and closely supervised physiotherapy.

Treatment preferences will vary between hospitals, and the A&E doctor should recognize that the injury is severe and refer to the orthopaedic team.

Initial treatment may consist of advice to elevate the limb, the application of a resting backslab (not a complete plaster), and to give crutches and analgesia.

For example, a Grade 3 tear to the medial collateral of the knee is a complete rupture and therefore permanent laxity of the ligament will be a major problem. The choice of treatment is between surgical repair or conservative methods. Total immobilization may be unnecessary but a brace must be used, such as the Lennox Hill and Don Joy varieties to prevent anteroposterior rotatory and valgus/varus strains being applied to the knee. The brace will also allow for continued flexion/extension movements, although full extension should initially be blocked with a hinge to allow the ligament to unite. Total immobilization will result in a tight scarred ligament that may be adequate. However, if the ligament is too tight then further trauma will occur when the joint is put under strain.

Nerve injury

Closed injuries to nerves may be due to compression, traction, and rarely to division of the nerve. Ischaemic injury may be important in the genesis of some nerve injury, especially in spinal stenosis.

Neuropraxia is the commonest closed nerve injury and is usually due to compression. The individual axons and neural bundles are in continuity and recovery is usually rapid and complete.

Axonotmesis occurs where there has been axon damage but microscopic structures continuing the axons (the endoneurium) are intact. The axons may thus regenerate along these channels and recovery usually occurs but takes much longer than a simple neuropraxia.

Neurotmesis occurs where the internal structure of the nerve is destroyed. This may be due to direct division of the nerve, but in musculo-skeletal problems the damage is more likely to be due to traction, prolonged compression, or ischaemia.

If the internal structure is destroyed then regeneration of the nerve will occur in a haphazard fashion and recovery is likely to be slow and, at best, incomplete. The more proximally a nerve is damaged then the poorer the recovery (e.g. brachial plexus injury).

Nerve lesions must be accurately diagnosed at the time of presentation, but this may be difficult. Sensation may be present (although it is always different) even in complete divisions of a nerve, and trick or mimicking movements may make the testing of motor function difficult. Any suspicion of nerve injury requires action and a more senior opinion.

Further reading

1. Alexander, R. M^cN. (1992). *The human machine*. Natural History Museum Publications, London.
2. Almekinders, L. C. (1996). *Soft tissue injuries in sports medicine*. Blackwell Science, Oxford.
3. Buckwater, J. A. (1994). Musculo-skeletal tissues and the musculo-skeletal system. In *Turek's orthopaedics. Principles and their application* (ed. S. L. Weinstein and J. A. Buckwater), pp. 13–68. J. B. Lippincott & Company, Philadelphia.
4. Hutson, M. A. (1990). *Sports injuries. Recognition and management*. Oxford University Press, Oxford.
5. Plattner, P. and Johnson, K. (1988). Tendons and bursae. In *The foot* (ed. B. Helal and D. Wilson), pp. 581–96. Churchill Livingstone, London
6. Renstrom, P. A. F. H. (1994). *Clinical practice of sports injury prevention and care*. Blackwell Scientific Publications, Oxford.

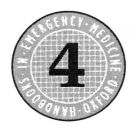

CHAPTER 4

Musculo-skeletal problems with no history of recent injury

Key points

- If there is no clear history of injury stop and think!
- There is a vast range of diagnoses in this group of patients.
- A full detailed history may be needed.
- Perform a general examination including temperature and pulse.
- Consider special tests such as white-cell count and erythrocyte-sedimentation rate.
- Before discharge consider — sepsis, ischaemic syndromes, referred pain, epiphyseal problems
- **S–O–F–T–E–R T–I–S–S–U–E–S** is an *aide-mémoire* to the causes of non-traumatic musculo–skeletal problems.

The range of diagnosis in non-traumatic musculo-skeletal problems

The spectrum of diagnoses in non-traumatic musculo-skeletal problems encompasses almost the whole of acute medicine. The misdiagnosis of these problems gives rise to complications that may be life- or limb-threatening. All medical students are taught that the limping adolescent with pain in the knee is the classical presentation of a slipped upper femoral epiphysis, but such cases are regularly missed in A&E departments. Shoulder pain is a 'classical' site for referred pain from the chest or abdomen but it may be disregarded with life-threatening results. The diagnosis of these conditions is difficult and often time consuming, but more time must be spent on these cases, just as there is an expectation to properly assess a case of chest pain.

A history noted to differ markedly from the typical arrests the listener's attention and puts him on his guard ... partly against a condition ... with which the physician is *so far* unfamiliar. (Cyriax)

Non-traumatic soft-tissue problems require careful detailed assessment

---

Some doctors might tend to label such patients 'inappropriate attenders'. This is a dangerous 'mind set'. While these patients may have sought medical advice from a more appropriate source the A&E department is duty-bound to assess these patients. While many patients will require referral back to their general practitioner for further investigation there is a clear responsibility to perform an adequate evaluation with the minimum of a good history and examination.

To think of a condition is often the first step in diagnosis. Many of the pathologies causing non-traumatic musculo-skeletal pain are rare and span most medical specialties, from genitourinary medicine to oncology, cardiology to dermatology. The scope is so great that throughout this book the acronym softer tissues will be used to provide a systematic framework to consider these problems.

In any given area certain pathologies will be highlighted but *any* of these categories may present with musculo-skeletal pain in *any* area of the body.

It might be argued that the diagnosis of many of these conditions is outside the scope of routine A&E practice. It is essential to exclude the life-or limb-threatening diagnoses such as sepsis, ischaemia, and referred pain. Many of the other conditions can be diagnosed using the basic clinical skills of taking a good history and examining the patient. If it is impossible to make a clear diagnosis the patient should be referred to their general practitioner or to an appropriate clinic.

Box 4.1 • Softer tissues: An acronym to aid the diagnosis of non-traumatic musculo-skeletal problems. 'To consider is to diagnose' applies in many of these conditions.

S — Sepsis
O — Osteoarthritis/degenerative disease
F — Fractures — stress, pathological, missed
T — Tendon, muscle, and deep bursae
E — Epiphyseal and childhood problems
R — Referred pain and neurological compression

T — Tumour
I — Ischaemia, imbalance of blood flow
S — Seropositive arthritides
S — Seronegative arthritides
U — Urate, calcium pyrophosphate and other crystal disease
E — Extra-articular rheumatism and endocrine and metabolic
S — Skin, fat, and subcutaneous bursae

Sepsis (Softer tissues)

Bacteriology, cellulitis, bursitis, abscess, osteomyelitis, septic arthritis, necrotizing fascitis

Bacterial infections

Of all infections presenting to A&E departments 90 per cent will be caused by either the Lancefield Group A streptococci (*Strep. pyogenes*) or *Staphylococcus aureus*. The majority of these infections are easily treated on an outpatient basis, but some patients will require admission to hospital either for surgical drainage of large abscesses, intravenous antibiotic therapy, or for treatment and investigation of some other rare, but more serious, infections such as septic arthritis, osteomyelitis, or necrotizing fascitis.

Staphylococcus aureus

These Gram-positive organisms are the cause of common septic lesions such as furuncles (boils), carbuncles, other abscesses, and osteomyelitis. More serious staphylococcal infections include septicaemia and toxic-shock syndrome.

The bacterium is resistant to penicillin due to its ability to produce beta-lactamase. Flucloxacillin is the drug of choice for community-acquired infections. Methicillin-resistant *Staphylococcus aureus* (MRSA) is an increasing problem in hospital practice and is beginning to emerge in community-acquired infections. This will pose an increasing problem for the treatment of staphylococcal infections in the future. Tetracycline may be used as some MRSA are still sensitive to this group of drugs. The alternatives, such as vancomycin, are mostly for intravenous, inpatient use only.

Erythromycin is the drug of choice in patients with a history of penicillin allergy. Clindamycin is an extremely useful antibiotic in all soft-tissue infections but has been associated with an increased incidence of pseudomembranous colitis. If this drug is used the patient should be reviewed on a regular basis and advised to stop therapy if diarrhoea or other gastrointestinal symptoms occur.

Group A streptococcus

Also known as *Streptococcus pyogenes* or the beta-haemolytic streptococcus, this Gram-positive coccus is a common cause of cellulitis and other spreading infections. The 'Group A' refers to the Lancefield group which depends on the type of polysaccharide surface antigens present on the organism. The group can be further subdivided into protein-antigen subgroups. These subgroups have different characteristics, some benign, some more invasive, some elaborate different toxins such as the erythrogenic toxin of scarlet fever, and some are more likely to produce autoimmune disease such as glomerulonephritis, rheumatic fever, or reactive arthritis.

Septicaemia, toxic-shock syndrome, and necrotizing fascitis are fortunately rare but devastating infections.

The organism is very sensitive to penicillin which is best given as ampicillin. Flucloxacillin is clinically effective against more minor streptococcal infections and can be used as prophylaxis. If the patient is allergic to penicillin then erythromycin should be used, or for severe infections clindamycin may be considered.

Rheumatic fever may present with musculo-skeletal pain and acute arthritis as an autoimmune disease after streptococcal infections.

Other bacterial infections

Anaerobic bacteria occasionally cause infections in wounds, especially following bites. It is standard practice to treat all animal bites and human bites with antibiotic prophylaxis. Co-amoxiclav (Augmentin) is effective against most of the bacteria causing such infections.

Sexually transmitted diseases are one of the most common causes of an acute monoarthropathy in young patients either due an acute septic arthritis (gonococcus) or reactive type arthritis (Reiter's disease).

Tuberculosis was becoming a rare cause of musculo-skeletal problems. However, there has been a increase in the prevalence of the disease in some countries associated with human immunodeficiency virus (HIV) infection.

Brucellois can cause acute arthritis or osteomyelitis.

Tetanus is a rare cause of wound infection due to high standards in wound cleaning and wound care, along with a national programme of tetanus immunization. However, 10–15 cases per year still occur in the United Kingdom.

Other clostridia may cause gas gangrene but this is rare in civilian practice. They are, however, sometimes grown as surface contaminants in chronic skin wounds such as pretibial lacerations. In this context it would be very rare to find the toxaemia of gas gangrene.

Lyme disease is a rare condition caused by the spirochaete *Borrelia burgdorferi*. It is transmitted by tick bites. It is a rare cause of arthralgia, myalgia, and arthritis. The presentation and difficulty in diagnosing this disease are vividly illustrated in a personal paper (see Vatrioyaara I).

Viral infections

Herpes simplex virus is the commonest cutaneous viral infection seen in A&E departments. Many cases are minor and self-limiting. Occasionally, this virus causes very painful local infection:

- herpetic whitlow (infection of the pulp space and paronychial region of the finger);
- herpetic stomatitis with ulceration of the gums and tongue as ophthalmic herpes;
- herpes zoster (shingles) is one cause of severe limb pain that can be difficult to diagnose. The pain precedes the rash and may mimic a whole host of soft-tissue problems, especially pain from a prolapsed intervertebral disc. Many minor viral infections require only symptomatic treatment.

Antiviral treatment (aciclovir) is indicated for more severe infections such as hepatic stomatitis, rapidly spreading infections, and hepatic whitlow. Suspected eye infection should be referred immediately to ophthalmology.

Sites of infection

Cellulitis

Cellulitis is an infection within the skin, normally caused by Group A streptococci. The signs are typical with a spreading, hot erythematous area, the area is tender.

Examination should include a search for sources of entry, palpation of local lymph nodes, and recording of the patient's temperature and pulse.

Minor episodes of cellulitis in healthy individuals may be treated on an outpatient basis. Intramuscular penicillin can be given at the time of visit and this can then be followed by an oral penicillin. If there is extensive cellulitis or if the patient is pyrexial or systemically unwell then they should be admitted to hospital for intravenous antibiotics.

Furuncles and carbuncles

These are infections of the hair follicles, usually caused by *Staphylococcus aureus*. The furuncle (simple boil) will normally respond to local measures such as bathing with warm saltwater.

It may require incision and drainage if there is fluctuation present. Antibiotics are indicated if there is spreading cellulitis.

Carbuncles are large abscesses, normally seen over the back of the neck, common in diabetics and other debilitated patients. This condition requires incision and drainage, the patient may require general anaesthetic and antibiotic treatment.

Bursitis

There are many subcutaneous bursae and a few deep bursae which are the common sites of inflammation. Only a minority of bursitis is caused by infection. However, it can be very difficult to differentiate between an *infective* bursitis and an *inflammatory* bursitis. Common examples are the prepatellar bursitis and infrapatellar bursitis of the knee and olecranon bursitis. This condition usually responds well to rest and anti-inflammatories, often antibiotics are given if the area is very red and hot and there is marked erythema. Very occasionally, incision and drainage is required.

Septic arthritis

This is an uncommon but severe cause of arthritis and must be excluded in any patients presenting with acute arthritis. There are 5 main causes of this condition:

- joint penetration
- haematogenous spread
- in joints fitted with prostheses
- following a therapeutic joint aspiration or injection
- a patient receiving steroid therapy.

Where there is a clear history of a penetrating injury (i.e. sole of the foot or knee) or where there has been medical intervention in or around the joint then the diagnosis is made easier. However, if there is no such history then the diagnosis can be very difficult. The patient presents with pain around the joint. The pain is severe and may keep the patient awake. The pain is worse on passive movement and there is restriction in movement in the 'capsular pattern'. Although the patient is often pyrexial with an acutely inflamed hot joint the classical signs of sepsis may not be fully established in the initial stages. Differential diagnoses include all the causes of acute arthritis, especially the acute crystal arthropathies. In such patients the joint should be aspirated and immediate bacteriological examination carried out. Patients with septic arthritis should be referred urgently to the orthopaedic team.

Septic tenosynovitis

The flexor tendons of the hand and foot are the commonest sites of this condition. There is often a history of a penetrating injury such as a cat bite or standing on a nail. Pressure in the sheath gives severe pain and extreme pain on passive stretch of the tendon.

Osteomyelitis

This condition is uncommon and becoming less common; for example, in a series of 100 children presenting with upper limb pain only one patient had osteomyelitis. The condition is becoming increasingly common in the elderly population, especially those who have had joint replacements.

The patient presents with pain, very often severe, there may be few cutaneous signs. However there is usually bone tenderness, X-ray is normal initially. The patient is usually pyrexial with elevated ESR (however, these may be normal).

In a child presenting with non-traumatic limb pain they should have a careful examination noting temperature, pulse, white-blood count, and ESR. If there are any signs of sepsis the child should be referred. Any child not using a limb should be reviewed within 48 hours. If the condition is not settling refer for a more senior opinion.

Necrotizing fascitis/pyogenic myositis

This is a rare condition due to invasive streptococcal or staphylococcal infection and has a high mortality rate. Early, aggressive surgery and antibiotic therapy are the mainstays of treatment for this condition. The initial symptoms may be vague and there may be little to find on examination apart from tenderness over the affected area. The patient is usually pyrexial. The condition may rapidly progress to a picture of a severely toxic patient. Clinical examination may be very misleading in that the main finding is severe pain over the affected sites. There may be swelling, but this is very subtle and erythema, if present, is very slight. The patient is pyrexial and tachycardic. An unwell patient with pyrexia and undiagnosed limb pain should have a more senior opinion.

Osteoarthritis and degenerative arthritis (sOfter)

The primary pathology in all osteoarthritis is the breakdown of normal cartilage function and structure. The most common causes for this is the normal ageing process, localized trauma such as intra-articular fractures or meniscal injury. Some individuals do appear to be more prone to the development of osteoarthritis as a more generalized disease.

Patients may present with long-term continuing osteoarthritic symptoms. They are more likely to present with an acute complication of the disease:

- acute joint effusions
- loss of function or movement due to loose body

- nerve root compression
- septic arthritis.

In an A&E department it is wise to exclude more serious causes of limb and joint pains before labelling the patient's symptoms as simply due to 'wear and tear'.

Fractures: stress, pathological, missed (soFter)

The main purpose of this text is not to review the detailed diagnosis and management of fractures but to bring to your attention that there are a number of fractures which must always come into the differential diagnosis of musculo-skeletal problems, even when the initial radiographs are normal.

Stress fractures

These occur when there is a sudden increase in activity or unaccustomed activity. The largest epidemiological series of these injuries are recorded in cohorts of military recruits undergoing training. The commonest sites are the 2nd and 3rd metatarsal shafts, the fibula, and the tibia.

History is typical with a sudden onset of pain, often following an increase in activity.

Examination reveals *specific* bony tenderness and pain on stressing the bone.

X-rays are normal for up to 3 weeks after the onset of symptoms.

Isotope bone scans can confirm the diagnosis if necessary, but in a typical clinical case the diagnosis can be made on history and examination. Patients need follow-up in the fracture clinic to ensure that the symptoms are resolving, and they usually do after 3–6 weeks.

Treatment is symptomatic, but a full explanation of the problem is required or patients may not rest properly.

Pathological fractures

Pathological fractures occur in the absence of significant trauma in a weakened area of bone. The commonest pathological fracture is the osteoporotic fracture of the vertebral body, but these may also occur in the feet and the tibia. More sinister causes, such as tumour or infection, also need to be considered in atypical presentations, especially if the pain is severe and night pain is a prominent feature.

Missed or old fractures

These may present with pain and swelling in the limbs with no definite history of *recent* trauma. The symptoms may be due to trauma some time in the past, but the effects only become manifest at a later date, examples of this would include trauma to the joint such as loose bodies within the knee joint or elbow joint.

Unfortunately, fractures can still be missed by A&E staff and/or may not be demonstrated on initial X-rays. The carpal scaphoid and small osteochondral fractures may be overlooked. It may take repeated examinations and even specialized tests such as a bone scan to diagnose these fractures.

Tendon and muscle problems (sofTer)

Tendon tears

Tendons may tear causing significant disability and loss of function. Examples include patellar tendon and flexor digitorum profundus tendon. The diagnosis of these conditions depends on demonstrating the loss of muscle function, especially on resisted movement. Other muscles in the same groups may mimic the function of a completely torn muscle and make demonstration of a tear more difficult. The best-known example for this is the persistence of foot plantar flexion in a complete tear of the Achilles tendon.

Tendonitis

Work-associated upper limb pain

Repetitive activity, or a sudden increase in the level of activity, undoubtedly causes soft-tissue problems. Conditions such as paratendonitis crepitans in a bricklayer have very clear histories and clinical signs. The phenomenon commonly known as 'repetitive strain injury' or 'tenosynovitis', however, is a complex problem and its diagnosis fraught with difficulties, both clinical and medicolegal. Inexperienced doctors in A&E departments should not use the blanket term 'tenosynovitis' to describe any upper limb disorder that may be associated with repetitive activity. Tenosynovitis is a very specific condition and should be used if there are definite signs of swelling over the course of a tendon sheath, pain on passive stretch of that specific tendon, and pain on resisted movement.

Acute paratendinitis

One of the most common, true-overuse syndromes is that of paratendonitis crepitans. This presents as a history of pain and swelling, pain on movement over the radial aspect of the forearm, usually following an episode of repeated activity such as hammering or digging. There are clear signs of swelling over the radial aspect of the forearm, along with tenderness at this site and characteristic crepitus on resisted extension of the wrist or thumb. Passive ulnar deviation is painful.

Other sites of paratendonitis include the extensors of the foot, just below the ankle joint.

Chronic paratendonitis

This is exemplified by tendonitis of the Achilles tendon. This condition is often more intractable to treatment and probably represents a combination of overuse and chronic degeneration. There is swelling around the tendon, local tenderness and pain on resisted movement. Other examples include the supraspinatous tendon at the shoulder.

Problems at the tendon/bone insertion

Enesthesiopathies

These occur at the attachment of muscles to bone. The best-known example is that of tennis elbow at the common extensor origin of the extensors to the humerus. The aetiologies of these conditions are complex, but overuse probably does have a significant part to play in their genesis. The main findings are pain and tenderness over the affected insertion, pain on resisted movement involving the muscle, and pain on passive stretch of the muscle.

Traction apophysitis

By definition, these are conditions of the growing skeleton. The commonest, best-known example is that of Osgood–Schlatter's disease where there is pain, swelling, and tenderness at the insertion of the patellar tendon to the tibial tuberosity. Any apophyses may be affected from the base of the 5th metatarsal through the apophyses around the knee joint, or around the pelvis especially the ischial apophysis.

Synchondrosis problems

Occasionally satellite ossification centres persist into adult life as 'normal variants'. The bipartite patella is an example where the two ossification centres are connected by a bridge of cartilage. Usually, these are asymptomatic, but occasionally overuse may lead to a chronic inflammation of the cartilaginous bridge. The diagnosis is made by a history of overuse, tenderness over the area, and a positive bone scan.

Epiphyseal and childhood problems (softEr)

Children are *not* small adults. While many of the conditions affecting children have their adult counterparts, there are a number of specific problems such as traction apophysitis (Osgood–Schlatter's disease), osteochondritis (e.g. Freiberg's disease), and epiphyseal problems such as a slipped femoral epiphysis (see Chapters 10, 11).

In the past, osteomyelitis and septic arthritis were commoner in children, but this is now changing with the ageing of the population and increasing numbers of surgical joint interventions.

Primary bone tumour, especially osteocarcinoma are commonest in the young and teenage age group.

Septic arthritis, slipped epiphysis, and bone tumours are rare, but it is understandable that missing these diagnoses causes considerable anxiety for both the child and parents and, occasionally, significant morbidity.

Referred pain and neural compression syndromes (softeR)

Referred pain

The missed diagnosis of referred pain can lead to very serious consequences. Common sources of referred pain include:

1. The spine, this may be due to true neural compression, as in true sciatica or cervical radiculopathy, or due to pain being referred from the facet joints of the spine.
2. From serious truncal pathology, classic examples include:
   - pain in the left arm due to cardiac pathology;
   - shoulder tip pain due to diaphragmatic irritation either from pneumonia or from intra-abdominal pathology such as a ruptured spleen;
   - leg pain due to aortic disease;
   - back pain due to aortic disease.

The diagnosis can be difficult, but the results of a missed diagnosis can be so catastrophic that referred pain should be considered where examination shows no evidence of local pathology at the site of the pain.

> **Referred pain must always be considered if there are no focal signs on examination of a limb or joint**

Neural compression

Compression or irritation of nerve roots due to spinal pathology is a very common cause of limb pain (sciatica, cervical radiculopathy).

There are a large number of peripheral neural entrapment syndromes and these are shown in Box 4.2. Median nerve compression is most common.

Box 4.2 • Nerve compression syndromes. Many are rare but radiculopathy, median, radial, and ulnar nerve problems are common

Upper limb
Cervical root radiculopathy
Thoracic outlet syndromes
Radial nerve
Posterior interosseous nerve
Ulnar nerve (at elbow and wrist)
Median nerve (above elbow, at elbow, at wrist)
Anterior interosseous nerve

Lower limb
Lumbar root radiculopathy
Meralgia paraesthetica
Obturator nerve
Common peroneal at knee
Tarsal tunnel
Morton's metatarsalgia.

Shingles

This can present difficulty in diagnosis. The symptoms are those of severe pain often in a dermatomal distribution that may be confused with nerve root compression or peripheral neural compression. The pain precedes the rash.

Tumour (Tissues)

The characteristic presentation is of pain, sometimes of a swelling. The commonest bone tumours are secondary deposits. Diagnosis is made by a history of pain which is often severe, swelling on examination (not always present), and on

X-ray appearances. The deposits tend to affect the more proximal skeleton including the ribs, spine, pelvis, femur, and
humerus. If such a diagnosis is made then an examination
should take place to exclude primary tumours in the chest,
breast, thyroid, kidney, and prostate.

Patients should be referred for appropriate further investigation and management.

Primary bone tumours are most commonly diagnosed in
children and teenagers, these range from benign bone cysts,
through to osteosarcoma. The patient may present early with
only a history of pain and no clinical signs. If X-rays are not
taken in A&E then patients should be referred to their general
practitioner for further investigation if these symptoms do not
improve after 1 week to 10 days.

Non-metastatic effects of tumours such as hypertrophic
pulmonary osteodystrophy may also cause musculo-skeletal
symptoms.

Ischaemia and vascular problems (tIssues)

*Vascular occlusion, vascular imbalance, compartment syn-
drome, Raynaud's disease, reflex sympathetic dystrophy*

Acute vascular occlusion/insufficiency

Lower limb pain with no history of trauma should always
prompt a careful examination of the arterial supply and
venous drainage of the lower limb. Intermittent claudication,
ischaemia and acute occlusion, and deep venous thrombosis
all present with limb pain. (This is further discussed in
Chapter X p. 000).

Compartment syndrome

Acute compartment syndrome usually occurs after trauma
although it can occur in the absence of trauma, for example if
there has been spontaneous bleeding into a compartment.
Severe unremitting pain with excruciating pain on passive

stretch of the affected muscle groups are the hallmarks of acute compartment syndrome (see Chapter X).

Chronic compartment syndrome may present with pain worsening on activity but settling with rest. It is caused by an increased compartment pressure due to slight muscle swelling during exercise (see chapter 12).

Raynaud's disease

This gives a characteristic clinical picture of digital vascular spasm, classically induced by cold. It can be induced by vibration and sometimes by soft-tissue vasculitis.

Reflex sympathetic dystrophy (Sudeck's atrophy)

This is an incompletely understood condition characterized by severe pain, skin changes, and osteoporosis. The skin is shiny red with increased blood flow. Treatment is likely to be prolonged and a senior opinion is essential.

Seropositive arthropathies (tiSsues)

This classically includes only rheumatoid arthritis, but in this book it will be taken to include all those causes of acute arthritis where there are measurable serum markers of auto-immunity such as rheumatoid factor, antinuclear factor.

These patients may present acutely to A&E departments either as a first presentation with an acute arthritis or as a complication of the disease.

Musculo-skeletal complications of rheumatoid arthritis include:

- septic arthritis
- tendon rupture
- joint subluxation/dislocation
- acute neural compression.

These patients will be known to the rheumatology team, therefore seek an early opinion, especially if there is a question that an acute joint effusion may be due to sepsis.

Seronegative arthropathies (tisSues)

This group of acute arthritis comprises a number of diverse conditions:

- ankylosing spondolysis
- arthritis with associated symptoms (Reiter's syndrome, arthritis plus inflammatory bowel disease)
- reactive monoarthritis
- rheumatic fever
- psoariatic arthropathy.

A detailed history gives the best chance of making a diagnosis of these conditions. Box 4.3 lists the questions to be asked of a patient with an unexplained joint swelling. The exclusion of joint sepsis is the main duty of the A&E department in these conditions, but early referral to the patient's general practitioner or the rheumatology clinic is advised.

Box 4.3 ● History in a patient with an acute monoarthritis

Any recent or past trauma
Any systemic upset, fever, rigors, vomiting
Any history of penetrating injury
Any previous similar joint swellings, either same joint or different joint
Any previous arthritis, if so which type
Any previous gout
Any previous history of back problems, inflammatory bowel disease, eye problems, skin problems, or genitourinary problems
Past medical history
Drug and alcohol history

Urate and calcium pyrophosphate crystal diseases (tissUes)

Acute gout and pseudogout are common. Patients attend due to severe pain and swelling. The commonest sites are the first metatarsal–phalangeal joint, small joints of the hand, subcutaneous bursae, and the knee.

Gout

Crystals of sodium urate in a joint cause acute gout. Crystals may also precipitate in the soft tissues as tophi and these can become acutely inflamed, mimicking a soft-tissue infection. There are many causes of high levels of blood uric acid, but the commonest associated problems in those presenting to A&E departments are alcohol and thiazide diuretics.

In an acute attack the patient, usually male, presents with a 24–48 hour history of increasing joint pain, swelling, and erythema. Examination confirms these symptoms along with signs of joint effusion and typical capsular pattern limitations in movement. The patient is apyrexial and systemic symptoms are uncommon.

Treatment with a non-steroidal anti-inflammatory will relieve symptoms dramatically (diclofenac 50 mg, 3 times per day for 3 days). Colchicine is an alternative (1 mg followed by 0.5 mg every 2 hours until the pain improves or side-effects develop up to a total dose of 10 mg).

The patient should be referred to their general practitioner for early review and future management.

Pseudogout (calcium pyrophosphate deposition arthropathy)

Calcium pyrophosphate crystals in a joint may excite an acute inflammatory response with a clinical presentation of an acutely swollen, hot painful joint.

The patient is usually elderly, the wrist and the ankle are most commonly involved. Systemic symptoms or fever are not usually present, but the condition may be hard to distinguish form septic arthritis. X-ray may show calcium deposition in the cartilages (chondrocalcinosis). Examination of joint fluid will show typical crystals.

Non-steroidal anti-inflammatory agents are the treatment of choice and the patient should be reviewed to ensure that symptoms are resolving.

Calcium pyrophosphate tendonitis

This is a common condition especially around the shoulder, but almost any tendon can be involved. Patients often present to A&E because of the acute pain. Tenderness is very localized and there are signs of a musculotendinous problem with pain on resisted movement or on passive stretch.

The diagnosis is confirmed by X-ray which shows the typical deposit of crystals.

This condition responds very well to injection with steroids and local anaesthetic (see Chapter 5 for technique).

Extra-articular rheumatism (endocrine and metabolic) (tissuEs)

This rare but important group of diseases affecting the soft tissues include a large group of connective tissue disorders such as polymyalgia rheumatica, dermatomyositis, and the extra-articular features of rheumatoid arthritis.

Polymyalgia rheumatica is mainly a disease of the elderly who present with significant pain and stiffness across the shoulder region. The ESR is raised and as such this is recommended as a screening test in any elderly person presenting with significant soft-tissue symptoms.

These conditions may well be difficult to diagnose in the A&E department and this is one of the major reasons for referring patients with undiagnosed musculo-skeletal problems to their GP for further assessment and investigation if necessary.

Endocrine and metabolic disease can have major effects on the skeleton. Osteoporotic fractures cause a huge amount of work in A&E. However, these diseases seldom present to A&E unless there are complications. However, Paget's, rickets, and osteomalacia may present with diagnostic problems.

Skin, subcutaneous fat, and bursae (tissueS)

Infection is the major problem affecting these areas, but overuse problems (callosity, bursitis) or inflammatory conditions such as bursitis are also common.

Skin rashes and nail signs are not uncommon in arthritic conditions. Gouty tophi, nail signs in psoariasis, rheumatoid nodules are but a few examples of diagnostic clues to be found on careful examination of the skin.

Further reading

1. Burgdorfer, W. and Schwan, T. G. (1996). Lyme disease. In *Oxford textbook of medicine* (3rd edn) (ed. D. J. Weatherall, J. G. G. Ledingham, and D. A. Warrel), pp. 689–91. Oxford University Press, Oxford.

2. Colman G. (1996). Pathogenic streptococci. In *Oxford textbook of Medicine* (3rd edn) (ed. D. J. Weatherall, J. G. G. Ledingham, and D. A. Warrel), pp. 497–510. Oxford University Press, Oxford.

3. Cyriax, J. (1982). *Textbook of orthopaedic medicine.* Vol. 1, Diagnosis on soft tissue lesions. Baillière Tindall, London.

4. Cyriax, J. H. and Cyriax, P. J. (1993). *Cyriax's illustrated manual of orthopaedic medicine* (2nd edn). Butterworth–Heinemann, Oxford.

5. Duerden, B. I., Reid, T. M. S., and Jewsbury, J. M. (1993). Soft tissue and eye infections. In *Microbial and Parasitic infection* pp. 306–18. Edward Arnold, London.

6. Espersen, F., Frimodt-Moller, N., Thamdurp Arrow, S., Dahl, V., Skinhoj, P., and Bentzon, M. W. (1991). Changing pattern of bone and joint effusions due to *Staphylococcus aureus*: A study of cases of septicaemia in Denmark 1959 until 1988. *Review of Infectious Diseases*, **30**, 347–58.

7. Eykyn, S. J. (1996). Staphylococci. In *Oxford textbook of medicine*, (3rd edn) (ed. D. J. Weatherall, J. G. G. Ledingham, and D. A. Warrel), pp. 523–32. Oxford University Press, Oxford.

8. Guidelines joint working group of the British Society for Rheumatology and the research unit of the Royal College of Physicians. (1992). Guidelines of a proposed audit protocol for

the initial management of an acute hot joint. *Journal of the Royal College of Physicians of London*, **26**, 83–5.

9. Klippel, J. H. and Dieppe, P. A. (1995). *Practical rheumatology.* Mosby, London.
10. Mubarak, S. J. (1993). Compartment syndromes. In *Operative orthopaedics* (2nd edn) (ed. M. W. Chapman), pp. 379–96. JB Lippincott, Philadelphia.
11. Paice, E. (1995). Reflex sympathetic dystrophy. *British Medical Journal*, **310**, 1645–7.
12. Verghese, G. (1996). Peripheral nerve compressions of the upper extremity. *The Orthopaedic Clinics of North America*, **27**.
13. Snaith, M. L. (1995). Gout, hyperuricaemia, and crystal Arthritis. *British Medical Journal*, **310**, 521–4.
14. Svenungsson, B. (1994). Reactive arthritis. *British Medical Journal*, **308**, 671–2.
15. Vatrioyaari

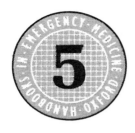

CHAPTER 5

Principles of treatment for soft-tissue trauma

Key points

- Give good advice preferably with written instructions.
- Use splints and crutches only for definite indications, if possible retain mobility.
- Analgesia:
  - paracetamol safe and effective;
  - non-steroidal anti-inflammatory agents may have some benefits where there are no contraindications;
  - little evidence that topical non-steroidal anti-inflammatory agents are effective in soft-tissue injury.
- Injections:
  - use and indications will depend on local departmental policy;
  - main indications are supraspinatus tendinitis and other calcific tendinitis, trigger finger;
  - other indications may require repeated injections;
  - subcutaneous atrophy may occur if the steroid is placed too superficially;
  - tendon rupture is a possibility.
- Physical treatment:
  - ice/heat readily available and effective but skin burns a possibility;
  - ultrasound/interferential by physiotherapist.
- Physiotherapy:
  - refer if severe injury but not requiring orthopaedic treatment;
  - moderate injury, but need to return to work/sport;
  - mild injury, but high functional demands;
  - specific injuries as outlined by local guidelines;
  - opinion and assessment if available immediately.

Introduction

It may be said that the majority of soft-tissue injuries heal 'in time'. However, the time factor may be of great importance both physically and mentally as well as psychosocially. The aim of treatment is to aid recovery and get the patient back to work and his sporting activities as soon as possible.

Treatment involves the treatment of an individual. To inform a keen runner that he has to rest due to an injury is inadequate. Equally, the main breadwinner for a family may not be able to afford a prolonged time off work.

Cursory advice just to stop exercise will result in a lack of trust between the doctor and the patient. Patients, and especially sports people, are taking an increasing interest in their bodies. The literature available to the lay-man today is extremely informative and therefore the medical profession must keep themselves up to date on exercise medicine.

The severity of an injury has a profound effect on treatment and rehabilitation. The site of an injury also has an influence. For example, compared to an upper limb injury, a lower limb injury may result in an inability to walk, go to work, etc. With long waiting lists for physiotherapy referral in some departments, the advice provided in A&E may be crucial in the first important days following a soft-tissue injury.

The main principle of treatment is to prevent the delay in healing and the harmful effects of scar tissue. The process of healing cannot be accelerated (although the patient may expect this). A too-early return to full activity may lead to an exaggerated inflammatory response, with a more prolonged and dysfunctional healing.

Chronic injuries caused by overtraining or overuse require an alteration in training techniques, for example the introduction of *cross training* (i.e. cycling will benefit a runner who shows early signs of a stress fracture), or an alteration in working practice. Once the injury is settling, then the patient is advised to return gradually to full activity.

External factors such as ill-fitting shoes, training purely on concrete, a racket that is too heavy all need to be addressed. *Internal* problems, overweight, smoking, poor nutrition, and poor flexibility will also be detrimental to the recovery of soft-tissue injuries.

Advice

Second only to accurate diagnosis, good advice is the most important part of the treatment of soft-tissue injury in the A&E department. The advice is not straightforward nor easily understood. Elements of the advice may appear to be conflicting, for example the patient may be confused that they are told to *rest* (initially) but then to *mobilize* and *use* the limb (after the acute inflammation phase).

The use of patient advice sheets is recommended and these may be easily produced for the more common problems (see the chapters on ankle, shoulder, elbow, and injuries knee). The advice should:

- explain the injury;
- give advice on the early treatment (RICE+ analgesia);
- give advice on rehabilitation exercises for flexibility, strength, and proprioception;
- give advice on action to take if recovery is prolonged or new symptoms develop.

An example of advice given for the ankle is shown in Box 5.1.

The patient may also require advice about work and driving. Patients should be told that they should not drive or operate machinery if they are not fully confident with the use of the injured limb.

Crutches and splints

Crutches

If a patient is unable to weight bear then crutches, a stick, or a walking frame will be needed. However, the prolonged use of crutches for a simple injury will greatly lengthen the rehabilitation period. The patient will have to be shown the correct way to use crutches, informed if they are to remain non-weight bearing, or if they should begin to partially weight bear as pain

Box 5.1 • Advice sheet (part of) for patient with a Grade 1 ankle sprain

You have sprained your ankle. This is a partial tear of one of the ligaments of the ankle joint. It is a painful condition but should slowly improve. You should be able to walk within 2–7 days (it will still be painful) and it may take 3–4 weeks to get back to full activity, even longer to return to full sporting activity.

In the first two days reduce the inflammation and pain by:
● Resting the injured limb;
● Applying ice for 10 minutes three times per day (wrap ice in towel);
● Wear support if given;
● Elevate the limb properly.

In the first two weeks slowly regain strength and function by the following types of exercises:
● Flexibility of the joint by stretching exercises (figure and explanation);
● Strength of the muscles (figure and explanation);
● Reflexes by balancing exercises (figure and explanation);
Do the exercises regularly (3–4 times per day).

After two weeks return to normal by gradually increasing your activity, for example:
● Once you can walk properly go for a gentle jog;
● Once you can jog increase the distance;
● Once you can jog well try running;
● Once you can run, try some of your work/sports activity, but not a competitive game;
● build up your activities slowly until you feel fit.

Getting worse rather than better? If you feel that progress is very slow or the pain and disability is getting worse then either contact your general practitioner or telephone the A&E department and we will make an appointment to see you again.

allows. Most patients will only need crutches for a few days; however, all should be reviewed either in the A&E clinic or the orthopaedic clinic. If they are still not weight bearing after one week then the original diagnosis should be questioned and appropriate arrangements made to rehabilitate the patient.

Bandages and splints

The choice of bandaging or splint will depend on local custom and practice, but it is important to use the appropriate method for each clinical situation and to be aware of the risks attached to these treatments.

Box 5.2 • Splintage. Match the type of splint to the therapeutic intention

Therapeutic intention	Method
Patient comfort in minor injury	Tubular bandage, elastoplast strapping
Patient satisfaction in minor injury	Tubular bandage, elastoplast strapping
Physical support of joint, retain mobility	Zinc oxide taping, functional bracing
Support for moderate/severe injury	Functional bracing, rigid splintage

---

Patient comfort and satisfaction in minor injury

Elasticated tubular bandages are often given to patients with minor sprains. However, it is unlikely that they give any significant physical support, although patients do seem to prefer some form of covering for the injured area. The patient should be instructed to remove the bandage at night, or if the limb swells, or if it becomes increasingly painful.

Elastoplast strapping or the use of wool and crepe bandaging are alternatives, but they only provide similar amounts of support.

Physical support in moderate injury

Taping The use of a proper taping technique can provide very good functional support for moderate sprains. However, the correct application takes skill and time and there are disadvantages, the most important being that the zinc oxide tape commonly used in these techniques does not stretch and if the taping is not properly applied there are increased risks of vascular compromise in a swollen limb.

Functional braces vary from simple wrap around elastic re-inforced material (e.g. eversion braces for ankle) to rigid hinged splints (Fig. 5.1). These are designed and reinforced to give support to specific structures while retaining joint movement.

Rigid support for moderate/severe injury

Functional hinged braces such as a knee brace provide rigid support to varus and valgus stress but allow flexion and extension.

Rigid plastic splints can provide short-term immobilization.

Metal reinforced material splints are widely available, and easily used (e.g. 'Futura' wrist splint).

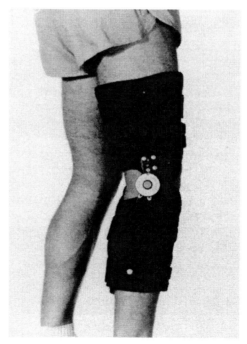

Fig. 5.1 ● Functional bracing. This allows joint mobility while protecting weakened structures. In this case there is free flexion/extension but the collateral ligaments are protected.

Plaster of Paris is the traditional method of immobilization. It is often used as a temporary splint for severe injury (usually as a 'back slab'). The main immediate complication is that of vascular compromise. Patients treated in Plaster of Paris must be given clear instructions to return immediately if they experience increasing pain, swelling, paraesthesia, or cyanosis of the limb. There is also a small, but important, risk of deep venous thrombosis in plasters applied to the lower limbs. The risks and benefits of this treatment should be considered. If a patient has a history of thromboembolic disease then seek senior advice before prescribing a lower limb Plaster of Paris.

Analgesia

Choice of analgesic

Analgesia is important for the treatment of any injury. There is still debate over the relative merits and risks of non-steroidal anti-inflammatory drugs (NSAIDs) in soft-tissue problems. There is a fine balance to be struck between the benefits of any treatment and the risks (Fig. 5.2).

Although NSAIDs are relatively safe, overusage for common problems will lead to a high number of side-effects. Paracetamol is a safe and effective analgesic and is recommended as a first-line analgesic for minor injury, especially in the elderly or if there are other contraindications.

For more severe injury, NSAIDs may be used in the young and fit. NSAIDs are the treatment of choice for acute inflammatory arthropathy, such as gout or pseudogout, and in such patients the undoubted benefits must be weighed against the risks.

Non-steroidal anti-inflammatory drugs in soft-tissue injury

These act as cyclo-oxygenase inhibitors blocking the production of prostaglandins and thromboxane from their precursor, arachidonic acid. By depressing the acute inflammatory response they lead to analgesia and decreased swelling.

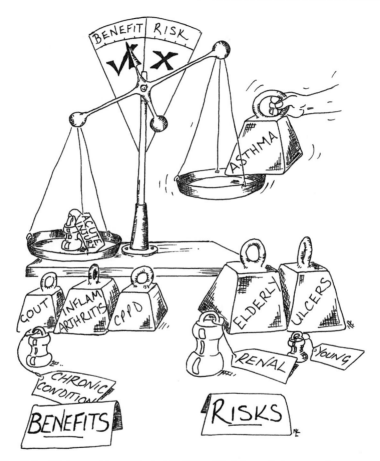

Fig. 5.2 ● Risks and benefits in NSAIDs. High benefit in crystal arthropathy and inflammatory joint disease. The marginal benefits in acute soft-tissue injury must be weighed against the significant risks in the elderly, peptic ulcer disease, and asthma.

Since acute inflammation is the normal reaction to soft-tissue injury there seems to be a logical argument supporting the use of these drugs. However, the evidence from clinical trials is less convincing. As stated above, judgement is needed to weigh the benefits against the risks. The contraindications to treatment include allergy, peptic ulcer disease, asthma, and in the elderly. The Committee on the Safety of Medicines (CSM) has issued clear advice over the use of these drugs.

'... in patients with a history of peptic ulcer disease and in the elderly, NSAIDs should be given only after other forms of treatment have been considered' and '... any degree of worsening of asthma may be related to the ingestion of NSAIDs' (see BNF ref.).

While there is some evidence that that topical NSAIDs are more effective than placebo in treating soft-tissue injuries, other studies have shown no benefits but a strong placebo effect. The use of these agents will depend on local departmental guidelines.

The effects of the acid secretion can be counteracted with the use of H_2 antagonists such as cimetidine (Tagamet 400 mg twice a day) or omeprazole (Losec 20 mg once daily). Prostaglandin analogues such as misoprostol (Cytotec 200 μg four times a day) have antisecretory activities thereby protecting the mucosa and allowing the ulcers to heal. These drugs may be used in combination with NSAIDS.

Which non-steroidal?

There are many NSAIDs and choice has to be made according to the differing therapeutic efficacy/side-effect ratios, pharmacokinetics, and the price of these drugs. Again the CSM has given clear advice on the relative risks of gastrointestinal haemorrhage due to NSAIDs. All the evidence seems to show

---

Box 5.3 ● Contraindications (some relative) for non-steroidal treatment

Allergy	warfarin
Elderly	anticonvulsants
Asthma	diuretics
Peptic ulceration	oral hypoglycaemics
Pregnancy	ACE inhibitors
Drugs	beta blockers

that ibuprofen (400–600 mg three times per day) is one of safest NSAIDs. Other drugs such as diclofenac (25–50 mg three times daily) or naproxen are second-line NSAIDs for the treatment of soft-tissue injuries or first-line drugs for the treatment of crystal arthropathies such as gout.

Corticosteroids and injection techniques

These drugs act as a phospholipase inhibitors. In A&E practice they have a few well-defined indications, but medical personnel do require training in the use of the techniques. Individual departments will have different guidelines on the use of steroid injections, but our experience is that they are most effective in painful conditions such as acute calcific tendinitis (e.g. supraspinatus tendinitis), stenosing tenovaginitis (e.g. trigger thumb). In enesthesiopathy (e.g. tennis elbow) they may give temporary relief of symptoms but may not be effective in the longer term. In other conditions, such as capsulitis of the shoulder there may be benefits in a course of 3 injections, but such a prolonged treatment regime is not usually the role of the A&E department.

Complications with the use of these drugs can be serious including sepsis, tendon rupture (after the inaccurate or injudicious use of steroid injection), and subcutaneous atrophy (if the drug is administered too superficially).

Warning If you have not been trained to give such injections seek advice and assistance from a senior colleague.

Technique

The exact point of injection is located and the skin marked if necessary. The patient is placed in the correct position and should be comfortable and fully informed of the procedure.

Sterile conditions are essential. The skin is cleaned with an antiseptic solution. Depo-Medrone or triamcinolone (40 mg/ml) is recommended and examples of the dosages are given in Table 5.1. A local anaesthetic may be mixed with the steroid solution.

Table 5.1 • Volume of Depo-Medrone (40 mg/ml stock solution) for specific sites

Site	Dose (mg)	Volume (ml)
Supraspinatus tendinitis	20	0.5–
Shoulder joint	40	1
Tennis elbow	20	0.5
Trigger thumb/finger	10	0.25

The location of the needle point is confirmed as follows:

- *Injection into a space such as a shoulder joint*   Try to aspirate some synovial fluid, the injection should meet with no resistance.
- *Injection into a tendon sheath*   Ensure that the needle is not in the tendon by asking the patient to gently move the tendon. Again the injection should meet with little resistance.
- *Injection into a lesion such as clacific supraspinatus tendinitis*   This is more difficult. There will be resistance to the injection. The aim is to give a number of 'micro-injections' to the lesion to spread the injection over the full area. The needle is moved by a tiny amount between each of these micro-injections. Spread of the steroid within the lesion may be encouraged by massaging the area for 2–3 minutes. The area of the injection site is covered.

The patient may develop an increase in pain (a crystalline flare) after a few hours and therefore they are advised to take regular analgesics for the first 24 hours after the injection.

The joint/area is rested for 1–2 days and the patient reviewed after 5–7 days. Repeated injections if used inapproriately may lead to long-term problems within the surrounding soft tissues (ligamentous laxity, degenerative joint collagen).

Supraspinatus tendinitis

1. Confirm the diagnosis.
2. Locate the **exact** area of maximum tenderness.
3. Mark this spot.
4. Use 0.5 ml (40 mg/ml stock solution of Depo-Medrone) and 1 ml of 2 per cent plain lignocaine.

5. Make sure the needle is very firmly attached to the syringe.
6. Go through the skin and into the inflamed lesion.
7. There will often be a grating sensation at the needle tip.
8. Give many 'micro-injections', altering the position of the needle by a minute amount after each push.
9. Massage the area for 2–5 minutes
10. Tell the patient to rest, that the pain may get worse, and to take some suitable analgesia.

Trigger thumb

1. Explain the technique to the patient.
2. Mark the spot of the tender nodule at the base of the thumb.
3. Use 0.25 ml of Depo-Medrone (40 mg/ml stock solution) and 0.5 ml of lignocaine.
4. Place the needle into the tendon sheath in the area of the nodule (check that the needle is not in the tendon by asking the patient to gently flex the IP joint of the thumb).
5. The injection should not meet with resistance, if it does, the needle is probably in the tendon, withdraw slightly and try again.
6. Massage the area.
7. Tell the patient to rest, that the pain may get worse, and to take some analgesia.

Physical treatment

Elevation

The correct methods of elevation are described in Chapter 3. These must be emphasized to the patient.

Cooling and thermal heating

Cooling

After a soft-tissue injury, heat should be avoided for the first 48 hours. The application of cryotherapy (crushed ice in a wet towel, frozen peas, ice massage, or a cryocuff mechanism which applies compression as well as cooling) should be applied for a maximum of 10–15 minutes as prolonged cooling produces a reactive vasodilatation. The aim is to produce local vasoconstriction and to reduce pain and swelling. Other effects include decreased nerve conduction therefore decreased pain plus a reduction in local temperature resulting in a fall in local metabolic demands.

The skin must be protected by a flannel or towel or burns may result. The application of an ice pack will cause some discomfort before the analgesic effect takes place. Contra-indications to ice therapy are: wounds; cold sensitivity (e.g. Raynaud's disease); and diseased skin lesions and peripheral vascular disease.

Superficial heat

This may be applied by various devices once the acute bleeding and swelling have subsided with the use of cryotherapy. Hot packs, rubefacients (liniment, e.g. 'Deep Heat'™) are inexpensive, easy to apply, and soothing. The manual application can also have a heating and analgesic effect (by providing a counterirritation stimulus and causing central inhibition of pain transmission, 'the gate theory'). Contraindications to heat are: bleeding; impaired sensation; malignancy. Some topical agents may cause skin hypersensitivity reactions.

Electrical stimulation

There are major gaps in the scientific evaluation, and hence understanding, of electrical stimulation and its effects. The benefits on dermal wound healing are proven and may therefore act as a model for the deeper soft tissues.

Ultrasound

Therapeutic ultrasound (1–3MHz) produced from a solid crystal applicator with an intensity range of up to 2 W/cm^2 can create a heating effect to a depth of 5 cm. Thermal effects are produced by continuous waves and are proportional to the amount of collagen in the tissue (i.e. maximal at bone/tendon junctions). Non-thermal effects (produced by both pulsed and continuous waves) are increases in blood flow, cell permeability, and protein synthesis. These are useful in the subacute phase. Contraindications are as for the thermal effects plus the application over epiphyseal lines, genitals, and false joints.

Interferrential

This applies an alternating current via two electric fields that are set to overlap at the chosen area. The effects have similarities to ultrasound plus a beneficial analgesic property by reducing swelling.

Galvanic/faradic stimulation (or iontophoresis)

With this method a direct current is passed into deeper tissues producing increased cellular activity and collagen synthesis.

Physiotherapy (and other specialist treatment)

When to refer?

The aims of **manual physiotherapy, osteopathy** and **chiropractice** are to restore ranges of movement and function to the musculo-skeletal system that the patient is unable to create unaided (e.g. due to pain, stiffness, lack of strength, or poor proprioception). The practitioners are often very experienced in the diagnosis and treatment of soft-tissue injuries.

The major problem is one of resources. If all musculo-skeletal problems were referred for physiotherapy then that department would be swamped. Consider physiotherapy if there is:

- severe injury;
- moderate injury, but a need to return to work/sport as early as possible;
- mild injury, but high functional demands (e.g. professional sports people, work needing high physical fitness);
- specific injury as outlined by local guidelines;
- an opinion on diagnosis and best treatment (if assessment is available at the time of initial attendance).

Patient assessment

The principles of assessment include all the history and examination details as recommended in this book; however, these practitioners often have greater training and experience of musculo-skeletal medicine than do many A&E doctors.

The complete evaluation of all the problems (biomechanical, physiological, structural, and functional) around the injured area requires such expertise. Types of evaluation include:

Isometric testing evaluates muscle power against resistance, the joint does not move and muscle length remains constant. This may be assessed manually (therefore only reliable on an intratester basis) or a hand-held dynamometer can be used.

Isotonic testing involves assessing the moving muscle and joint complex.

Isokinetic testing requires complex equipment with a constantly adapting device when the patient moves a joint. The equipment measures the forces developed during the movement and gives reproducible data that can monitor progress in rehabilitation.

Proprioceptive testing is a useful clinical test to assess the individual's ability to return to weight-bearing exercise. Balance training and postural awareness are essential to lower limb injuries. Static tests are often adequate for detecting the ankle that is prone to recurrent inversion.

Functional testing evaluates the performance of the patient, as a whole, in a complex activity and is an essential part of evaluating fitness to return to sport or work.

Psychological assessment 'Half the cure is wishing to be cured.' Good therapists, like good doctors, try to treat the patient as an individual, taking account of the psychological response to injury. Failure to appreciate these responses may lead to a breakdown in confidence and motivation. The classic phases are: denial immediately after injury; bargaining ('surely I can be back in 2 weeks rather than 4?'); depression; and finally acceptance (when the most constructive functional rehabilitation can begin). Involvement of the patient in decision making should be part of the support system.

Treatment

During the initial stages of injury the aims are to reduce pain and swelling using the physical treatments listed above (e.g. ice, electrical stimulation). Some early movement is encouraged, although this may need the protection of strapping or a brace rather than total immobilization in a cast which, if not indicated, will be detrimental to the vital first few days and weeks of treatment.

Physiological and biomechanical normality is the aim of treatment to prevent the problems of recurrent injury or stress to an area distal to the initial injury. Failure of rehabilitation will affect the whole kinetic chain of movement. For example, a javelin thrower with a knee injury may plant the injured limb incorrectly. Due to the altered transmission and absorption of forces through this area, the thrower will have to compensate elsewhere to produce the required performance. Hence, a lower back or shoulder injury will often occur with poor rehabilitation of a lower limb injury in throwers.

Supervised exercise regimes

The therapist will be able to advise and supervise an individual programme of rehabilitation structured to the patient's requirements. Such regimes commonly have three elements:

• strength training;
• stretching and mobility training;
• proprioceptive training.

The emphasis on the type of training will depend on the injury, for example in a neck sprain most of the exercise will be directed at posture and regaining mobility, while in an ankle sprain all three types of training are important.

During injury, maintenance of fitness should not be forgotten. For example, with knee injuries, swimming with a pool buoy and cycling both maintain cardiovascular performance. Cycling with the unaffected leg has benefits in the maintenance of muscular development in the affected limb.

Manual treatments

Manipulation Reduction of dislocations and subluxations will normally be carried out by medical staff. However, manipulation may be required to break down adhesions that are preventing joint mobility.

Mobilization This term implies a more gentle and controlled process than manipulation. The aim is to restore joint mobility.

Massage and friction These techniques produce pain relief through the same process of counter-irritation as that produced by the use of rubefacients.

Summary

- Treat the injury.
- Mobilize and restore function as soon as possible.
- Prevent re-injury.
- Maintain fitness of other systems.
- Aid sport-specific rehabilitation.
- Provide psychological support.

Further reading

1. Anon. (1995). Articular and periarticular corticosteroid injections. *Drugs and Therapeutics Bulletin*, **33**, 67–70.
2. *British National Formulary* (1995). British Medical Association and The Pharmaceutical Press, London.
3. Campbell, J. and Dunn, T. (1994). Evaluation of topical ibuprofen cream in the treatment of acute ankle sprains. *Journal of Accident and Emergency Medicine*, **11**, 178–82.
4. Corrigan, B. and Maitland, G. D. (1994). *Musculo-skeletal and sports injuries*. Butterworth–Heinemann, Oxford.
5. Cyriax, J. H. and Cyriax, P. J. (1993). *Cyriax's illustrated manual of orthopaedic medicine* (2nd ed). Butterworth–Heineman, Oxford.
6. Griffin, L. (1995). *Rehabilitation of the injured knee* (2nd ed). Mosby, St Louis, Missouri.
7. Grigg, P. (1994). Peripheral neural mechanisms in proprioception. *Journal of Sport Rehabilitation*, **3**, 2–17.

8. Houglam, P. (1992). Soft tissue healing and its impact on rehabilitation. *Journal of Sport Rehabilitation*, **1**, 19–39.
9. Hutson, M. A. (1990). *Sports injuries recognition and management.* Oxford University Press, Oxford.
10. Kennedy, J. C. and Baxter Willis, R. (1976). The effects of local steroid injections on tendons; a biomechanical and microscopic correlative study. *American Journal of Sports Medicine*, **4**, 18–21.
11. McLatchie, G. R. *et al.* (1985). Variable schedules of ibuprofen for ankle sprains. *British Journal of Sports Medicine*, **19**, 203–6.
12. Anon. (1994). Rational use of NSAIDs for musculo-skeletal disorders. *Drugs and Therapeutics Bulletin*, **32**, 91–5.
13. Renstrom, P. A. F. H. (1994). *Clinical practice of sports injury prevention and care.* Blackwell Scientific Publications, Oxford.

CHAPTER 6

The shoulder joint

Key points

- Normal range of movement — flexion 160 degrees, extension 50 degrees, abduction 170 degrees, adduction 50 degrees, internal/external rotation 70 degrees;
- Capsular pattern — limitation in abduction/external rotation and internal rotation in extension (arm up behind back);
- Very mobile units with lax capsule — main factors maintaining stability are the rotator cuff muscles;
- Acromioclavicular joint injury — common, may be a total dislocation of the joint;
- Supraspintous tear — is a common injury, may need operative repair in young person;
- Anterior dislocation — usually easily diagnosed and treated, but exclude major fractures and nerve/vascular injury;
- Posterior dislocation — epileptic fits and electric shocks usually cause this injury **Easily missed**;
- Traumatic effusion — common in the elderly, recovery is often prolonged and incomplete (1–2 years);
- **Consider referred pain — myocardial infarct, pneumonia, intraabdominal pathology.**

Anatomy and mechanics

The shoulder is capable of more movement than any other joint. It is susceptible to a wide range of acute and chronic soft-tissue injuries. The powerful and well-coordinated musculature around the shoulder has an effective shock-absorbing action. An overriding external force is more likely to dislocate the shoulder or fracture the clavicle than result in a bony injury to the humerus or glenoid (except in elderly people and in children who sustain fractures of the upper humerus). Fractures more commonly occur at the wrist, elbow, humerus, and clavicle.

The shoulder *joint* is the glenohumeral joint. However, the shoulder *girdle* consists of four other joints: the acromioclavicular (ACJ), sternoclavicular (SCJ), scapulothoracic, and subacromial joints. Movements of the shoulder often involve the whole of the shoulder girdle, therefore when examining any one part of this complex it is important to isolate the exact joint you wish to test.

The glenohumeral joint is a shallow 'ball and socket', the glenoid cavity is deepened by the fibrocartilaginous glenoid labrum. The articular area of the glenoid is only one-third that of the humeral head. The capsule of the joint is lax, especially inferiorly where there is minimal muscular tissue (further reasons why this is the most common joint to dislocate). Anterior capsular thickenings, the coracohumeral and transverse humeral ligaments provide a little support. The main joint stabilizers are the rotator cuff muscles (supraspinatus, infraspinatus, subscapularis, and teres minor (Fig. 6.1).

Shoulder movements and biomechanics

The axis of the joint passes medially as the arm is brought forwards. Flexion of the limb therefore involves some adduction at the shoulder. Lateral rotation occurs above 90 degrees of abduction to prevent impingement of the humeral head on the acromion. The throwing action consists of cocking (abduction, external rotation, and extension), acceleration (adduction, internal rotation, and adduction), and follow-through (where

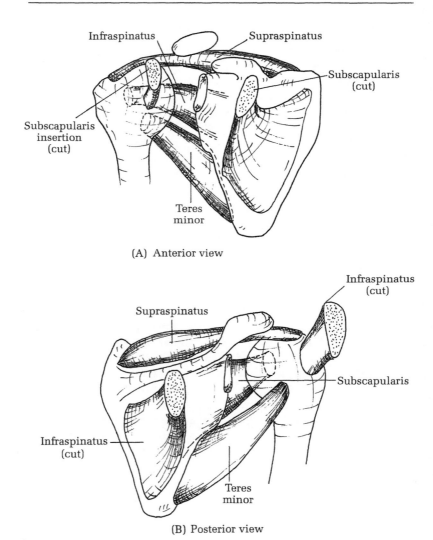

(A) Anterior view

(B) Posterior view

Fig. 6.1 ● The rotator cuff. (A) Anterior view (thorax removed!) Subscapularis inserts to the lesser tuberosity and is a major anterior stabilizer. (B) Posterior view. The other three muscles insert into the greater tuberosity.

deceleration forces have to be controlled by the rotator cuff). This complex biomechanical mechanism is very susceptible to injury. Once the balance of the shoulder has been affected, adaptations may take place leading to further trauma.

Examination

Both shoulders, clavicles, and upper chest are fully exposed.

Joint above — Begin examination by checking neck movements and the sternoclavicular joint.

Look — Observe from both the front and back. Look for deformity, steps over the ACJ, any signs of swelling.

Feel — Carefully palpate the SCJ, clavicle, acromion, scapula, head of the humerus, upper humerus, and elbow.

Move — Isolate the glenohumeral joint by placing a hand over the ACJ and restrict scapulothoracic movement.

Check if a capsular pattern is present (limited external rotation/abduction/internal rotation in extension).

Check if there are signs of a painful arc on abduction.

Check active abduction from neutral (to ensure rotator cuff is not completely torn).

Nerves and vessels — Check axillary nerve function by testing sensation over the deltoid insertion. Check radial, median, and ulnar nerve function. Check the pulses and **compare** in both arms.

In non-trauma check the vital signs, examine the neck, and consider chest/abdominal examination

---

Trauma — fall on to the shoulder

ACJ injury, supraspinatus tear, traumatic capsulitus

History

The commonest history is of a simple fall but beware of higher energy injuries such as falls from heights or high-speed road traffic accidents. Symptoms are usually of notable discomfort at the superior aspect of the joint plus mild discomfort at the point of impact over the deltoid region. Movements are all painful apart from rotation in neutral which is relatively pain-free.

Level of activity has to be taken into account. Any restricting lesion around the shoulder will limit the sports person or the manual labourer.

Examination

Joint above — Ask the patient to move their neck through the range of movement.

Look — Compare with the other side and observe elevation and swelling of the ACJ. The deltoid bulge is preserved indicating that the GH joint is located. The arm is held in adduction.

Feel — Commence around the SCJ and proceed proximally. Try to locate the exact areas of maximum tenderness. Gentle depression of the ACJ will invoke discomfort confirming the site of the pathology. Palpation should include the scapula and then the tendinous structures the rotator cuff and biceps tendon.

Move — The degree of active movements will be restricted especially those involving abduction, elevation, and end-of-range rotatory movements. Passive movements will be just as restricted if the ACJ is injured. Gentle resisted movements will cause little pain. The ACJ may be stressed by placing one hand on the midclavicle and pressing upwards, axially along the humerus (Fig. 6.2). Specifically check abduction. If this is absent then consider a complete rotator cuff tear.

Investigations

X-ray the shoulder and/or the clavicle as indicated. The SCJ is very difficult to image on plain X-ray, if there are significant signs around this joint CT may be required. Specific views of the ACJ include comparison views of the other ACJ or weight-bearing views that may show increased joint space on the affected side if ligamentous disruption has occurred. Chest X-ray may be needed if there is an associated chest-wall injury.

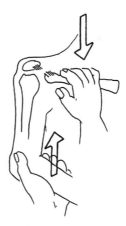

Fig. 6.2 ● Stress testing the ACJ. Stabilize the clavicle and apply proximal compression through the flexed elbow.

ACJ–SCJ injury

Sternoclavicular joint injury These are uncommon. Anterior subluxations and dislocations are treated as for ACJ injury. Posterior dislocations may cause serious damage to the upper airway or the great vessels at the root of the neck. Refer immediately.

Acromioclavicular joint Ligament injury to the ACJ may vary from a Grade 1 sprain to complete disruption (Grade 3). Initially rest in a broad arm sling, advise ice and analgesia. Total dislocation will result in 4-weeks restricted-movement advice followed by a gradual return to full function. A therapeutic strapping may be applied to temporarily compress the joint.

Subluxed joints may be mobilized under careful observation once the initial symptoms have resolved. Refer unstable ACJ injuries or dislocations to the fracture clinic.

Rotator cuff tears

These can be partial or complete and can be very disabling, especially in young, fit individuals. Large tears may require surgical repair and accurate diagnosis is needed.

History

The history is of a severe blow to the shoulder, for example in a rugby tackle or in a road-traffic accident. A fall on to the outstretched hand may also cause this injury.

Examination

There is usually little swelling or bruising at the time of presentation. There is specific tenderness just below and anterior to the tip of the acromion. Pain is maximal on active abduction. Rotations are relatively free. A classical painful arc is hard to demonstrate in the acute tear due to severe pain. Resisted abduction is painful and weak indicating a partial tear. Active abduction may be absent indicating a complete tear.

Investigation

X-rays are normal.

Treatment

Rest in a broad arm sling initially, but give the patient every encouragement to mobilize the arm. Arrange a review, especially in young patients with significant mechanisms of injury. If after 2–3 weeks there are still major symptoms then orthopaedic review is indicated and further investigations such as arthography may needed. A large tear in a young person probably merits surgical repair.

Traumatic effusion

History

Falls on to the arm or shoulder often result in bleeding or lead to an effusion within the shoulder joint. In the elderly this may lead to a stiff painful shoulder with a similar clinical course to adhesive capsulitis. The patient (usually more than 50 years of age) often presents 4–10 days after a fall with pain and severe limitation of movement.

Examination

Look — There is no deformity, the patient often supports the damaged limb and undressing is difficult.

Feel — There is generalized tenderness around the upper humerus.

Move — Active and passive range is restricted in the 'the capsular pattern', with restriction of lateral rotation (both active and passive) restricted more than abduction, which is more limited than internal rotation (unable to put an arm up their back or to comb their hair).

Investigation

X-rays are taken since a fracture of the surgical neck of the humerus is common, if the upper humerus is in three of four parts refer to orthopaedics.

Treatment

Early mobilization is essential. Distraction physiotherapy techniques may be employed. Chronic lesions at this site can cause long-term morbidity therefore review by general practitioner or physiotherapist is advised.

Trauma — dislocated shoulder

Anterior dislocation

The patient often presents with the diagnosis already made (by the patient, relative or paramedic). The younger the patient the greater the incidence of recurrent dislocation becoming a problem, as the anterior capsule and glenoid labrum may fail to reattach properly (the Bankart lesion).

History

The force is overriding (e.g. during a submission hold in judo) or instantaneous as in a fall (such that the patient has no time to react). A previously dislocated shoulder requires surprisingly little provocation to recur especially after poor rehabilitation. If the presentation has been delayed (more than 12 hours) reduction may be more difficult. Beware long-standing 'dislocations' in elderly patients or patients with stokes, attempts at reduction often fail. Arrange orthopaedic clinic review.

Examination

Look — The arm is held in adduction and internal rotation. There is concavity in the deltoid area due to the absence of the humeral head (compare with the other side).
Feel — Start the examination lower down the upper limb or by palpating the other shoulder. Gentle palpation will confirm the findings of observation. Check for bony tenderness of the clavicle and shaft of humerus.
Move — The patient will be unwilling to allow either active or passive movement. It is unnecessary to move the limb if the diagnosis has been made. **Nerves and vessels** — Check axillary nerve sensation and deltoid movement. Check the median and ulnar nerve. Check the pulses.

Investigations

Radiographs of the area should be taken to confirm examination findings and to exclude a major fracture. If there is a fracture of the humerus then refer to orthopaedics for reduction.

Treatment

The dislocation must be reduced. There are various manoeuvres described but many can be performed with ease; gentle movement, care, and time taken to overcome muscle spasm are the keys to success. Analgesia such as entonox and an opiate may be given. Sedatives such as midazolam may be needed, but **take great care** if mixing an opiate and midazolam. Respiratory arrest is not uncommon after such a combination and it is preferable not to use these drugs in combination.

You should be trained to reduce a shoulder by an experienced senior but the modified Kocher manoeuvre is described (Fig 6.3).

1. The patient must be relaxed and in the supine position, give opiate analgesia or midazolam. Entonox may also be used.

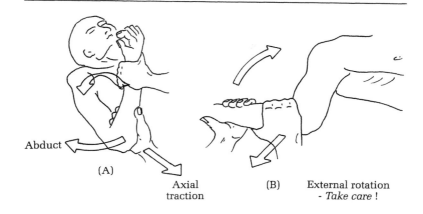

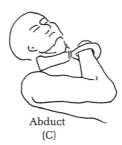

Fig. 6.3 ● Reduction of anterior dislocation. (A) Gently abduct the arm while applying gentle axial traction. (B) Externally rotate, be gentle this manoeuvre may cause a fracture. (C) Adduct and internally rotate the shoulder.

2. Talk to the patient to provide further distraction and relaxation.
3. Gently abduct the arm while gently applying increasing axial traction. An assistant may apply countertraction to the humeral head which may be felt in the axilla.
4. As maximal abduction is reached, gently externally rotate the shoulder. Do not use undue force at this point as the arm is now acting as a long lever and humeral fracture is possible.

5. If reduction has not been achieved by this time adduct the arm while internally rotating.
6. After relocation, immobilize by a body bandage and broad arm sling. Re-check the nerves and vessels.
7. **X-ray again to confirm reduction** and arrange for review in the fracture clinic.

Posterior dislocation

History

This is the key to diagnosis and this condition should be excluded in any patient with shoulder pain following an electric shock or an epileptic fit.

Examination

There is seldom any visible deformity, although the head of the humerus may be visible below and lateral to the point where the spine of the scapula joins the acromion. All movements are painful and restricted. Check neurovascular function.

Investigation

X-ray — Failure to obtain the correct films is the main reason for missing this injury. It can be very difficult to perform an axillary view as the patient is unable to abduct the arm due to pain. Alternative views include the lateral scapular view. The 'light bulb sign' (Fig. 6.4 A,B) can indicate posterior dislocation, but this appearance may be due to a normal rotation of the head of the humerus.

Treatment

If a patient cannot move the shoulder after a fit or shock arrange for review.

If a posterior dislocation is diagnosed then refer to orthopaedics.

Pitfalls

1. Missed fractures.

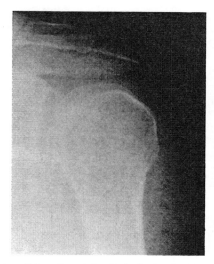

Fig. 6.4 • Posterior dislocation: The 'light bulb sign' is caused by rotation of the humeral head. It is often seen even when the shoulder is in joint.

2. Missed posterior dislocation.
3. Failure to establish full movement due to delayed rehabilitation.
4. Damage to the subclavian vessels/brachial plexus/axillary nerve.
5. Poor shoulder mechanics due to rotator cuff injury.

Non-trauma — severe pain (SOfTeR tissues)

Sepsis, Capsulitis, tendinitis, bursitis, referred pain.

History

An accurate, detailed history is needed. The pain could be due to **life-threatening** problems such as myocardial infarct or a ruptured ectopic pregnancy. The onset, progress, and type of pain is documented, as are associated symptoms (see page 25).

Examination

General — The patient may look unwell and in pain. The pain of acute tendinitis, capsulitis, and bursitis may be severe and keep the patient awake. Check the temperature, pulse, and blood pressure.

Joint above — Check the range of movements of the neck.

Look — There is often little to see. **If swelling is present then this is unusual** — think of sepsis, tumour, or a rarer condition.

Feel — The area over the shoulder may be warm. If it is hot then think of sepsis. In supraspinatus tendinitis the tenderness is very specific, just below and anterior to the tip of the acromion.

Move — In *adhesive capsulitis* there is a typical 'capsular pattern' of restricted movement — marked reduction in external rotation, abduction, and internal rotation in extension. Resisted movements are relatively pain-free. In *supraspinatus tendinitis* rotation is spared, but abduction is very painful beyond 60 degrees. There may be a typical painful are where abducting the arm causes pain between 60 and 100 degrees, but above this the movement is relatively free. **Resisted abduction** is painful. In *subacromial bursitis* the findings are similar to those of supraspinatus tendinitis, but as the muscle/tendon is not involved, resisted abduction in neutral is relatively pain-free.

If there are no signs of local shoulder pathology with full range of movement, examine the neck, chest, and abdomen

---

Nerves and vessels — Check the pulse, motor, and sensory function of the main nerves.

Investigations

X-ray may show calcification within the supraspinatus tendon confirming the diagnosis. ESR or white-cell count may be indicated. Other investigations such as ECG or chest X-ray may be indicated by clinical assessment.

Diagnosis and treatment

Sepsis (Softer) — Pyomyositis is a very rare variant of necrotizing fasciitis where the muscles themselves are the site of infection. The large muscles around the shoulder are one of the commonest sites for this condition. Diagnosis is difficult in the early stages, but the warning signs are of severe pain, a pyrexial patient, muscle tenderness and pain on passive stretch of the muscles. Septic arthritis/osteomyelitis occasionally presents in the shoulder.

Adhesive capsulitis (sOfter) — Adhesive capsulitis (frozen shoulder) is a painful and disabling condition. The cause is unknown but it may be a type of inflammatory arthritis or an acute response to joint degeneration. The patient is usually over 60 years of age. They present with pain and limitation in movement.

Examination — The joint may be slightly warm. Tenderness is diffuse. There is a classical limitation of movement in the capsular pattern (limited abduction/external rotation/and internal rotation in extension.)

Treatment — Early mobilization and active physiotherapy may prevent long-term stiffness. Cortico steroid injections reduce the length of the disability, but, since they need to be repeated such treatment is probably outside the responsibility of the A&E department. The patient is given advice to exercise the shoulder (leaning forward with the arm hanging and making circular movements with the arm and abduction exercises), analgesia, and referred to their general practitioner.

Tendon, muscle, bursa (sofTer) — Subacromial bursitis — The bursa provides a cushion between the rotator cuff muscles and the humeral head. Repetitive active movements (swimming, cricket, baseball) cause impingement within this area that will also be exacerbated by inflamed tendons and resultant swelling. The pain is often felt in the deltoid region with discomfort when lying on shoulder.

Examination typically reveals a *painful arc* on abduction between 60 and 100 degree but no pain on resisted abduction in neutral.

Treatment Injection therapy may be indicated if the pain is severe and the patient is seen soon after the onset of symptoms. The condition usually spontaneously resolves within 14 days.

Rotator cuff tendinitis

The supraspinatous muscle reinforces the superior aspect of the joint capsule prior to insertion of the greater tuberosity of the humerus, producing shoulder abduction. The tendon is subject to repeated traumas and compression by the coracoacromial arch. This may lead to minor injury that may heal abnormally (e.g. by heterotopic calcification, mucoid degeneration) or the tendon may tear partially or completely. This pathology leads to the clinical syndrome of supraspinatus tendinitis, a common condition that presents frequently to A&E departments.

Examination The main findings are of localized tenderness over the rotator cuff, and pain on specific resisted movements (Table 6.1).

Treatment Acute calcific supraspinatus tendinitis is one of the few problems where steroid injection is definitely indicated in the A&E department. The condition is so painful and the relief so definite that it is recommended. The technique is outlined in Chapter 5. For other lesions or where the diagnosis is not certain then rest, non-steroidal anti-inflammatory agents, and physiotherapy are indicated.

Biceps tendinitis — This presents as anterior shoulder pain and pain on lifting/elbow flexion. There is tenderness over the tendon (between the lesser and greater tuberosities) with pain

---

→

Fig. 6.5 ● Signs of shoulder instability. (A) Sulcus sign. This is demonstrated by downward distraction of the upper arm on the fixed shoulder. If inferior instability is present a sulcus appears below the acromion. Produced with permission from Wallace and Hutson *Sports Injuries*. Recognition and management. Oxford Univ Press 1991.
(B) Anterior apprehension test. The shoulder is held in 90 degrees of abduction and external rotation. Apprehension will occur in the abnormal joint, when the humeral head is forced anterior by the examiner's hand placed behind the patient's upper arm.

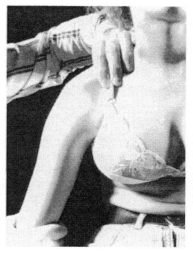 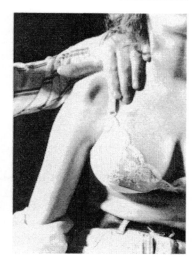

(A)

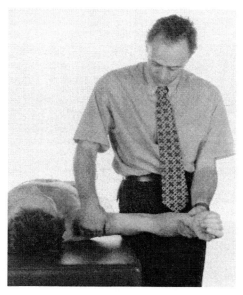

(B)

Table 6.1 • Findings in tendinitis of individual parts of the rotator cuff

Tendon	Pain	Restricted movement
Supraspinatus	Anterior/deltoid	Abduction (painful arc)
Infraspinatus	Posterior deltoid	Lateral rotation
Subscapularis	Anterior/deltoid	Medial rotation/adduction
Teres minor	Scapular	Lateral rotation

on resisted elbow flexion and supination. Treatment by physiotherapy or injection of steroid may be required.

Chronic instability/subluxation — This is commonly seen in middle-aged and elderly patients, probably as a late result of previous trauma. It is also seen in patients with hemiparesis in whom the joint may actually dislocate. Athletes may also have similar problems.

The complaints are of pain and clicking on movement and a feeling of instability. The apprehension tests and the sulcus sign may give clues to the nature of the instability (Fig. 6.5). Further investigation and treatment may require CT, MRI, or arthroscopy.

Referred pain (softeR) — The treatment is wholly dependent on accurate diagnosis. While shoulder tip pain is regarded as one of the 'classical' sites of referred pain, diagnoses of cardiac, chest, and abdominal pathology are easily missed. Where the patient looks unwell and has severe pain then examine the chest/heart/abdomen and cervical spine. Arrange a chest X-ray or ECG if indicated.

Pitfalls and how to avoid them

- Supraspinatus tears — if patient is unable to actively abduct then arrange orthopaedic clinic review.
- Complete A–C joint dislocations — if suspected arrange orthopaedic clinic review.
- Posterior dislocation — suspect in any epileptic fit/electric shock — ask for appropriate X-rays.
- Referred pain from chest/diaphragm — always suspect if very few local signs in shoulder.

Further reading

1. Commission on the Provision of Surgical Services. (1993). *Guidelines for sedation by non-anaesthetists.* Royal College of Surgeons of England, London.
2. Crenshaw, A. H. (1992). Shoulder and elbow injuries. In *Campbell's operative orthopaedics* (ed A. H. Crenshaw), pp. 1733–1768. Mosby Year Book, St Louis, Missouri.
3. Hutson, M. A. (1990). *Sports injuries recognition and management.* Oxford University Press, Oxford.
4. Kay, N. R. M. (1989). The painful shoulder — diagnosis and treatment. *Rheumatology in Practice,* **7**, 20–6.
5. Kessel, L. (1982). *Clinical disorders of the shoulder.* Churchill Livingstone, Edinburgh.
6. Perry, J. (1993) Biomechanics and functional anatomy of the shoulder. In *Operative orthopaedics* (2nd edn) (ed. M. W. Chapman), pp. 1641–50 J. B. Lippincott, Philadelphia.
7. Poppen, N. K. (1993). Soft tissue lesions of the shoulder. In *Operative orthopaedics* (2nd edn) (ed. M. W. Chapman), pp. 1651–72 J. B. Lippincott, Philadelphia.
8. Ticker, J. B. and Bigliani, L. U. (1995). The coracoacromial arch and rotator cuff tendinopathy. *Journal of Sports Medicine and Arthroscopy Review* (New York), **3**, 8–15.

The elbow joint

Key points

- The joints of the elbow (including the proximal radioulnar joint) have strong ligaments. The main movements of the elbow joint are flexion and extension while forearm pronation and supination occur at the radioulnar joints.

- Trauma
  - Fractures are common but may be hard to detect on X-ray leading to a misdiagnosis of a soft-tissue injury. (Especially radial head fractures and children's fractures.)
  - The presence of a traumatic effusion within the elbow joint often indicates an occult fracture.
  - The fat-pad sign is one of the most useful soft-tissue signs in musculo-skeletal radiology (see Fig. 7.3).
  - Severe ligament injuries are often misdiagnosed.
  - A 'pulled elbow' (subluxation radial head from the annular ligament) is a common presentation in a toddler.

- Non-trauma
  - Acute swelling over the point of the elbow is often due to olecranon bursitis.
  - Pain in the elbow on lifting may be due to a number of mechanical problems, but tennis elbow is the commonest (inflammation at the origin of the wrist extensors).

Anatomy and biomechanics

The elbow consists of the radio-humeral, ulnar-humeral, and superior radio-ulnar joint. The joints are strengthened by the radial collateral, ulnar collateral, and annular ligaments. As with many joints the strength of the associated musculature is the main supportive structure in resisting forces applied across the upper limb. Hyperextension forces may cause impingement signs in the ulnar-humeral space (pain at the back of the elbow on extension, limited extension). Damage to the annular ligament is often misdiagnosed as an acute tennis elbow and occurs following a forced end-of-range movement in pronation or supination.

The elbow appears to be at its greatest risk when involved in a closed kinetic chain (the distal limb is fixed or taking weight) sport such as gymnastics and contact sports such as judo.

Movements and biomechanics

The ulnar/radio-humeral joints act as a hinge allowing flexion and extension. The superior radioulnar joint is of the pivot variety and is involved, along with the radiohumeral joint, in pronation and supination.

The normal ranges of movement are shown in Fig. 7.1. Flexion, 135 degrees; extension, 0 degrees; pronation, supination, 180 degree range.

Examination

Joint above — Ensure that there is no tenderness over the clavicle and that there is good range of movement of the shoulder.
Look — The patient with significant joint injury is often holding the elbow in a typical way with the elbow flexed to about 70–80 degrees and the forearm in a midrotated position. Note any swelling, deformity, or bruising. Bruising may not be evident for for 2–3 days, and by this time it can be very marked spreading down the arm to the wrist.
Feel — Note the points of maximum tenderness and palpate all the bony landmarks.

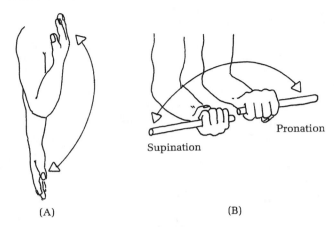

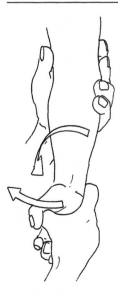

(A)   (B)

Fig. 7.1 ● Ranges of movement at the elbow joint. (A) Flexion until the forearm contacts the arm; extension 180 degrees. (B) Rotation, keep elbow flexed and close to body to exclude shoulder movements; range 180 degrees.

Fig. 7.2 ● Pulled elbow reduction. Supinate and extend the elbow.

Move — The typical capsular pattern is of limitation in extension, flexion, and rotation, but the most obvious deformity is the limitation in extension.

Nerves and vessels — Always check the pulses very carefully and check the ulnar, median and radial nerve.

Investigations

X-ray — The standard views are anteroposterior and a true lateral. Obliques of the radial head may be required to confirm small crack fractures.

Trauma

Pull on arm in child

History

This is a common presentation. The toddler (1–4 years of age) sustains a 'pull' along the arm (e.g. parent pulling on arm when the child stumbles). The child cries after the incident and then will not use the arm. The child is otherwise well with no other symptoms.

Examination

Joint above — Check the clavicle and shoulder.
Look — The child is reluctant to move the arm but there is no swelling or bruising.
Feel — Palpate the whole limb from clavicle to wrist, there is usually no tenderness.
Move — Elbow flexion and extension may be normal but often there is some limitation of extension. Forearm rotation, especially supination, is painful.

Investigations

X-ray is not required in a typical case with a good history and relief of symptoms on manipulation.

Treatment

The elbow is grasped with the thumb over the radial head. The other hand holds the child's hand and extends and fully supinates the forearm, (Fig. 7.2). This usually reduces the subluxation. If this fails, the situation is explained to the parents and the child is brought back for review in 2 days. By this time they are often using the elbow normally. If not, then further opinion is advisable.

Trauma — fall on outstretched hand

Fracture radial head, dislocation, medial ligament rupture, pull of medial epicondyle

Falls on the outstretched hand often lead to an elbow injury. Fractures of the radial head, the olecranon, and epiphyseal injuries in children can be difficult to diagnose. A significant history and a swollen stiff elbow suggest moderate to severe injury. X-ray and follow-up is advised.

With this mechanism of injury the whole of the limb is at risk. Examine from the clavicle to the wrist as an initial screening test (see Upper limb screening test, p. 132).

History

The magnitude and direction of force are important is assessing these injuries. Pain and loss of movement are the main symptoms.

Examination

Joint above — Move the neck through the full range of movements. Check shoulder movements and palpate down the arm.
Look — Compare the elbows, noting any swelling, bruising, and the way the limb is held at rest.
Feel — Palpate the key bony landmarks.
Move — Gently move the elbow through the passive range. *Loss of full extension signifies a joint effusion.* Pain on forearm

rotation indicates radial head/or radial neck injury. Stress the collateral ligaments gently (elbow flexed 20–30 degrees). Test resisted power of biceps, triceps, and wrist flexors/extensors **Nerves and vessels** — Neural and vascular injury are common. Check: radial pulse, radial nerve, ulnar nerve, and median nerve.

Investigations

Standard X-ray views should be taken, radial head obliques may be indicated if there is a high suspicion of fracture but none is visualized on the initial films. Difficult fractures to diagnose are shown in Fig. 7.3A.

Children's radiographs are often difficult to interpret. Seek advice. If the child's elbow is very swollen comparison films may be needed, but these should not be routine.

The finding of a fat-pad sign is very significant

A fat pad (Fig. 7.3B) indicates a haemarthrosis and is usually caused by a fracture such as the radial head or an undisplaced supracondylar fracture.

Treatment

All significant displaced/comminuted fractures should be referred to the orthopaedic team. If no fracture is seen but there is a positive fat-pad sign then the patient is advised that they may have a fracture but that no fracture is visible on the X-rays, they are given a collar and cuff sling, and an analgesic. Review is arranged in the A&E department or in the fracture clinic depending on local guidelines.

Significant soft tissue injuries with marked swelling and limitation in movement are given a collar and cuff and advised to **gently** mobilize the joint. Forced extension should **not** be used. *Myositis ossificans* is a troublesome late complication of elbow injury and may be exacerbated by a too-rigorous mobilization. Review is required for moderate/severe ligament injury with marked swelling and limitation of movement.

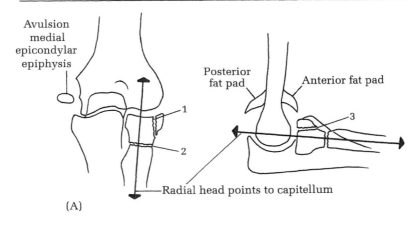

Avulsion medial epicondylar epiphysis

1
2

Radial head points to capitellum

(A)

Posterior fat pad

Anterior fat pad

3

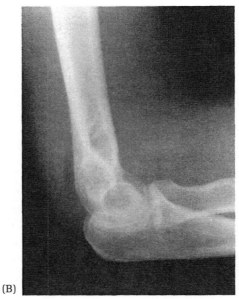

(B)

Fig. 7.3 • Anterior and posterior fat pad signs indicate acute elbow joint swelling. Commonly missed injuries include fractures of the radial head (1), radial neck (2), the coronoid process (3) and in children avlusions of the medial epicondylar epiphysis. Dislocation of the radial head is excluded by ensuring that the radial head points to the capitellum in all views.

> **Elbow routine** — the elbow is rested in a collar and cuff but the patient is told to take the arm out of the sling for 5 minutes in every hour and to gently flex and extend the elbow. They must not force the elbow straight and only work within the limits of pain. As the pain improves then the period of exercise can be extended

Children with significant pain or swelling or loss of function should be reviewed by someone with experience within 2 days (see below). Significant injury is easy to overlook in the child's elbow.

Review

At review a careful history would be taken and examination would note any tenderness over the clavicle and shoulder and any restriction in shoulder movement. The *exact* points of tenderness (e.g. distal humerus, medial epicondyle, radial head) would be sought by gentle palpation. The restriction in movement would give important clues (e.g. pain on pronation/supination indicating a radial head problem). The X-rays would be scrutinized noting the alignment of the bones, especially the radial head (should always point to the capitellum). Bones are examined in detail, especially those areas highlighted in Fig. 7.3A, comparison views may be required. Cartilaginous areas of the growth plates are examined and soft-tissue signs such as anterior and posterior fat-pad signs are excluded. A radiologist's opinion may be requested and if there is marked swelling an orthopaedic opinion requested.

Dislocated elbow

History

The history is usually of a fall. The deformity is obvious. Check the radial pulse, and the function of the radial (posterior interosseous), median, and ulnar nerves.

Investigations

X-rays are needed before reduction to ensure that there are no fractures. The humerus lies anterior to the radius and ulna and there may be lateral displacement. Common associated fractures are of the radial head and the coronoid process of the ulna.

Treatment

Adequate sedation or analgesia or a general anaesthetic are required. With the elbow flexed to 20 degree, axial traction is applied to the forearm against counteraction. While maintaining the traction any lateral displacements are corrected and the elbow is further flexed. Clinically, the reduction can be confirmed by flexing the elbow fully and also by checking the relationship of the bony landmarks (see above). The radial pulse and neurological function are rechecked. Reduction is confirmed by a check X-ray and the arm rested in a collar and cuff beneath clothes. Follow-up is arranged in the fracture clinic.

Traumal — pitfalls and how to avoid them

- *Missed elbow effusion on X-ray.* Check the lateral view very carefully and exclude appearances such as those shown above.
- *Missed avulsion of the medial epicondylar ossification centre.* The patient is a child with a significant fall and pain and swelling most marked on the medial side of the elbow. Look carefully at the medial epicondyle and the joint space. If necessary obtain views of the other elbow. Refer to the orthopaedic team if you suspect this injury.
- *Missed radial head/neck fracture* Do not ignore the classical clinical presentation of pain and limitation of extension and supination along with X-ray signs of an elbow effusion.
- *Failure to appreciate severe medial collateral ligament injury.* The elbow is very swollen. Bruising may take a few

days to appear. The signs are most marked over the medial side of the elbow, with pain on valgus stressing of the joint.
• *Development of myositis ossificans.* Heterotopic calcification in the muscles anterior to the joint is not uncommon. Avoid vigorous early mobilization (see Elbow routine box) If an elbow injury appears to be getting worse during the first 10 days take steps to verify that the diagnosis is correct (? X-ray again? Further views? Orthopaedic opinion?)
• *Missed radial head dislocation.* Examine for signs of fracture of the ulna. Check that the radial head points a the capitellum on all views.

Non-trauma — pain and swelling around elbow (softer tiSsUeS)

Olecranon bursitis

The condition may be caused by repeated minor trauma or leaning on the elbow. It is usually inflammatory, but occasionally a single direct blow may cause a sudden bleed into the joint. Gout and rheumatoid arthritis may cause a similar clinical presentation. However, some cases are due to infection and it can be very difficult to distinguish between the causes on clinical examination alone.

Examination

Look — There is a large red swelling over the point of the elbow with an appearance of a spreading cellulitis.
Feel — The area is hot and very tender. The swelling is fluctuant.
Move — There is normal elbow extension indicating that the joint is not involved.

Treatment

The initial treatment is rest and a non-steroidal anti-inflammatory agent. If there is significant erythema then give antibiotics (flucloxicillin 250 mg for 10 days).

Organize review by the GP within 1–2 days.

Aspiration may be needed and occasionally incision and drainage is required if the condition appears to be worsening in spite of rest and antibiotics or if the lesion appears to be 'pointing'. A sample should to sent to microbiology and antibiotics prescribed.

Non-trauma — pain on lifting and moving (sOFTER tissUes)

O, osteoarthritis; F, missed fractures; T, tennis elbow, golfers elbow, biceps problems; E, osteochondritis dissecans; R, ulnar nerve entrapment; U, gout

Assessment

History

The exact onset and type of symptoms are recorded. A history of **locking** or inability to extend are important pointers to intra-articular problems such as loose bodies.

Examination

Feel — Exact point of tenderness are palpated. In tennis elbow the area of the lateral epicondyle is the most painful area.

Move — Limitation of active or passive range in the 'capsular pattern' or lack of full extension and flexion indicate an intra-articular problem such as a loose body, or joint effusion.

Resisted wrist movements are the key to diagnosis in tennis and golfer's elbow (Figs 7.4A,B).

Nerves — Examine the functions of the ulnar, radial, and median nerves in detail.

Osteoarthritis (sOfter)

Previous trauma, fractures, and osteochondritis will lead to osteoarthritis which is noted on X-ray and is demonstrated by bony restriction at the end of range of all elbow movements. There is seldom pain. Flare of a mild synovitis can be treated with NSAIDs. Flexibility and strength of the musculature can be improved by physiotherapy. Loose bodies and the occasional obstructing exostosis can be referred for operation.

Fractures (soFter)

Difficult fractures are shown in Fig. 7.3A. Intra-articular lesions such as osteochondritis dissecans may be located by a C.T. scan if suspected with the typical 'loose body' history in the teenager.

Tendon and muscle problems(sofTer)

Medial and lateral epicondylitis are common overuse injuries. The history is of pain on lifting or gripping. There may be a history of recent overuse or a direct blow.

Biceps tendonitis can cause anterior elbow pain. Pain occurs with active resisted flexion and supination. Passive pronation may also impinge the inflamed area.

Triceps or biceps may rarely be avulsed from their insertions (there may be a small avulsion fracture). Weakness and pain on resisted movements suggest this diagnosis. Unlike ruptures of the muscle belly (see p. 43) Avulsions of the insertions of these muscles may require surgical repair, especially in a young, fit individual.

Biceps muscle may rupture, usually at the junction of the belly and the proximal tendon of origin. The patient presents with bruising and pain and there is an obvious lump in the arm on resisted elbow flexion. Treatment is rarely indicated.

Examination

Look — There is seldom any swelling or bruising.

Feel — There is local tenderness at the origin of the wrist extensors from the lateral epicondyle (tennis elbow) or the wrist flexors at the medial epicondyle (golfer's elbow).

Move — Active resisted wrist movement confirms the diagnosis as will passive stretch of the muscles (Fig. 7.4).

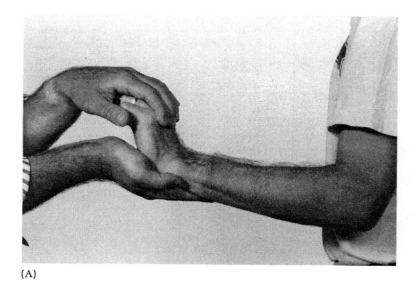

(A)

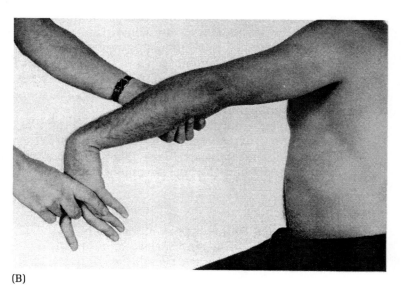

(B)

Fig. 7.4 • Tennis elbow. Pain on (A) resisted wrist extension, and (B) on maximal passive stretch confirm the diagnosis.

Treatment

This consists of avoiding the aggravating factors, adjusting sporting equipment (e.g. weight and handle size of tennis racket) and correcting poor work practices. Specific braces may be used. Local steroid injections may be helpful, but the patient is best referred to the general practitioner for these continuing treatments.

Epiphyseal and childhood problems(softEr)

Osteochondritis dissecans may present with symptoms of a loose body (locking and lack of extension). Young gymnasts are at risk of radiohumeral injuries since the closed kinetic requirements of their work involve extension and compression of the elbow. X-ray is required and may show the osteochondral defect, the loose body, or an elbow effusion. Refer these cases to the orthopaedic department.

Referred pain and neural compression (softeR)

The ulnar nerve is very susceptible to compression as it winds around the medial epicondyle.

The median nerve may be compressed as it passes through the two heads of the pronator muscle. The symptoms are of tingling in the hand and fingers in the sensory distribution of the affected nerves. There may be some weakness. Tapping over the nerve may cause the symptoms. If there has been no recent injury then refer the patient to their general practitioner for further investigation and follow-up.

The anterior and posterior interosseous nerves may also be compressed at or below the elbow. These are motor nerves and weakness or clumsiness may be the presenting complaint. Detailed examination may show weakness of the flexor pollicis longus and the superficial flexors to the index and middle fingers (anterior interosseous) or of the thumb extensors (posterior interosseous).

Note

If there are no signs around the elbow then the upper limb as a whole should be examined. Pain commonly radiates from the shoulder, wrist, and neck.

Further reading

1. Apley, A. G. and Solomon, L. (1995). *Apley's system of orthopaedics and fractures* (7th edn). Butterworth–Heinemann, Oxford.
2. Corrigan, B. and Maitland, G. D. (1994). *Musculo-skeletal and sports injuries*. Butterworth–Heinemann, Oxford
3. Cyriax, J. H. and Cyriax, P. J. (1993). *Cyriax's illustrated manual of orthopaedic medicine* (2nd edn). Butterworth-Heineman, Oxford.
4. Gellman, H. G. (1992). Tennis elbow. *Orthopedic Clinics of North America*, I, **23**, 75–81.
5. McRae, R. (1990). *Clinical orthopaedic examination* (3rd edn). Churchill Livingstone, Edinburgh.
6. Wadsworth, T. G. (1982). *The elbow*. Churchill Livingstone, Edinburgh.

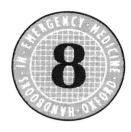

The wrist

Key points

- Anatomy
  - The area of the wrist comprises a complex series of joints including the distal radioulnar joint.
  - The joints are highly mobile and dependent on strong ligaments for stability.
- Trauma
  - Fractures of the scaphoid are one of the commonest missed diagnoses in A&E practice. Be reluctant to label an injury as due to 'wrist sprain' in a young patient with pain or swelling in the wrist after a fall or other significant injury. Such patients require senior review within 14 days.
  - Falls on the hand in a child may result in fractures anywhere along the limb and these may be difficult to localize and diagnose. Seek senior review of a child not using a limb.
  - Ligament injury may cause significant long-term disability.
- Non-trauma
  - Fracture of the scaphoid may present late with pain, swelling, and instability. X-rays are recommended. Osteochondritis of the lunate is a rare cause of similar problems.
  - Beware the diagnosis of 'tenosynovitis'. True tenosynovitis is an uncommon condition. Paratendinitis crepitans and De-Quervain's stenosing tenovaginitis are more common and both have very specific signs.
  - Median and ulnar nerve compression both above and at the wrist are common causes of non-traumatic wrist and hand pain.

Anatomy and biomechanics

The wrist is a complex area encompassing the distal radio-ulnar joint, radiocarpal joint, the intracarpal joints, and the carpometacarpal joints. The joints are highly mobile and their stability and function are highly dependent on strong intact ligaments. Therefore ligamentous damage ('wrist sprain') may result in significant long-term symptoms and disability. The mobility also results in a precarious blood supply to some of the carpal bones, for example the scaphoid. Damage to this blood supply may result in poor healing of fractures or avascular necrosis.

The wrist joint movements take place mainly at the joints between the proximal and distal carpus (except ulnar deviation which is a radiocarpal joint movement). The scaphoid acts as a 'bridge' across the proximal and distal rows and thus is the site of major stresses in forced hyperextension, hyperflexion, and some rotational injuries (fracture scaphoid, scapholunate ligament tears, carpal dislocations).

The carpometacarpal and the intrametacarpal joints allow little movement except the specialized thumb carpometacarpal joint (see Chapter 9).

Examination

Joint above — Falls on to the outstretched hand may transmit forces up the entire limb and can result in a whole series of injuries. Routinely, commence examination with the elbow, but in children, the elderly, or if there are proximal symptoms then begin with the clavicle and work distally.

Look — Locate the points of maximum swelling. The swelling may be very subtle, especially in the 'anatomical snuff box' (ASB). It is essential to compare the limbs.

Feel — In patients with localized wrist symptoms begin commencing palpation at the elbow (except in children or those patients with poorly localized symptoms, commence examination at the neck). Palpate the radial head, the humeral epicondyles, and then continue down the length of the radius and ulna. Wrist palpation must be accurate and localized. The important landmarks are shown in (Fig. 8.1).

Move — A quick and easy screening for the whole of the upper limb is shown in Figs 8.2 A–C This, along with specifically testing full elbow extension excludes significant injury to the shoulder girdle and elbow joint. (However, **beware** of **non-traumatic** causes of pain.) Test pronation and supination. Pain on this movement suggests injury to one or both of the radioulnar joints.

X-ray — Unless the injury has been very trivial, X-ray is indicated. The standard views of the wrist are the anteroposterior and true lateral views.

> **If there is any tenderness or swelling over the scaphoid request specific scaphoid views**

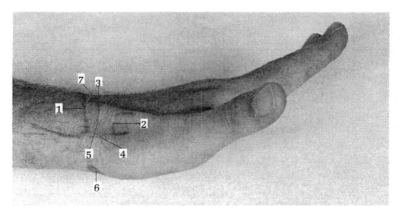

Fig. 8.1 ● Surface anatomy of the wrist. 1, Distal radius; 2, 1st metacarpal base; 3, tendon of extensor pollicis longus; 4, tendons of extensor brevis/abductor longus; 5, scaphoid; 6, scaphoid tubercule; 7, dorsal wrist joint.

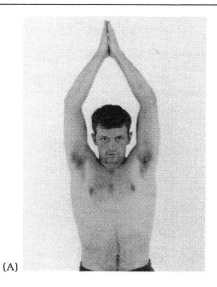

(A)

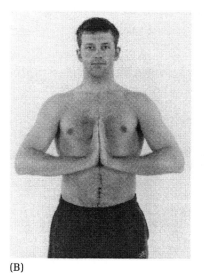 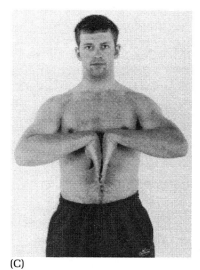

(B)   (C)

Fig. 8.2 • Upper limb screening test. (A) Shoulders fully abducted, elbows extended. (B) Wrists and fingers fully extended elbow flexed. (C) Wrists fully flexed.

Trauma — fall on outstretched hand

In patients between 15 and 50 years of age

Fractured scaphoid, other carpal fractures, ligament injury, triangular cartilage injury (see also Chapters 6 and 7)

History

The commonest mechanism is a hyperextension injury. The symptoms are of pain, swelling and loss of function.

Examination

Joint above — Always examine the elbow/forearm.
Look — Compare both wrists carefully. Swelling in the area of the anatomical snuff box is indicative of a scaphoid fracture. Swelling over the dorsum indicates a wrist effusion.
Feel — Examine the elbow and radial head. Palpate down each of the forearm bones, the distal radioulnar joint, the anatomical snuff box, the scaphoid tubercule, the carpal bones, and the metacarpal bases.
Move — Active and passive movements are limited. Note whether pronation and supination are affected indicating damage to the distal radioulnar joint/triangular cartilage. *Axial compression* along the line of the first metacarpal compresses the scaphoid. Ask the patient to grip.
Nerves and vessels — Examine the function of the median and ulnar nerves and capillary refill.

Investigations

Good quality X-rays are essential in the assessment of wrist injury. One serious error is the failure to obtain proper radiographs in scaphoid injury. If there is tenderness in the area of the scaphoid then request specific scaphoid views, these include anteroposterior, a true lateral, an oblique, and anteroposterior taken in maximal ulnar deviation.
Other specific views such as carpal-tunnel views may be needed for rarer fractures such as those of the hamate.

Interpretation

A, Alignment — Ensure that there is normal carpal alignment (Figs 8.3 A–D). Confirm the correct relationship of the 'three Cs' of the distal radius, lunate, and capitate. If this is not checked then serious carpal dislocations will be missed and the injury treated as a 'sprain'.

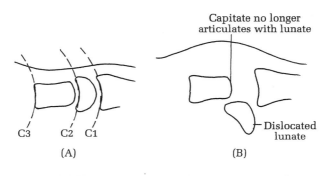

Capitate no longer
articulates with lunate

C3   C2   C1

Dislocated
lunate

(A)   (B)

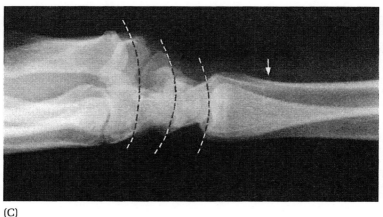

(C)

Fig. 8.3 ● Carpal alignment. Check the position of the 'three C's'. The distal radial articular surface (C1), the lunate (C2), capitate (C3) should all be in the correct position (A,C). A normal pronator fat pad is seen (arrow). Carpal dislocations: the alignment of the 'three C's' is lost (B,D).

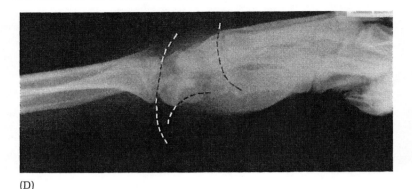

(D)

Fig. 8.3 • Continued

B, Bones — Trace each of the bones in turn, difficult fractures are highlighted in Fig. 8.4. The major problem is the scaphoid. Often 'scaphoid lines' can be seen, these may or may not be a fracture. Treat on **clinical** grounds as described below.

C, Cartilage — Check the spaces between each of the bones, these should be equal. A large gap (more than 0.3 cm) between the lunate and the scaphoid may indicate a significant intracarpal ligament injury.

S, Soft tissues — Swelling in the wrist joint is indicated by bulging over the dorsum on the lateral view (Fig. 8.4). This sign indicates significant wrist pathology. Also the pronator quadratus fat pad can be seen as a radiolucent line lying anterior to the distal radius. The distance from the periosteum to the pad should be less than 10 mm, (Fig. 8.4).

Treatment (Fig. 8.5)

> **Always ensure that a fracture of the scaphoid has been excluded. This may require several visits in patients with tenderness over the scaphoid**

There is no test, either clinical or radiological, that can exclude a scaphoid fracture at the first visit. Indeed it may be

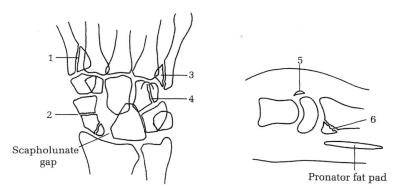

Fig. 8.4 ● Difficult wrist fractures. Soft-tissue signs of dorsal swelling and a pronator fat pad distance of more than 1 cm indicate acute wrist swelling and significant intra-articular injury. 1, Bennet's; 2, scaphoid; 3, metacarpal base/dislocation; 4, hamate; 5, avulsion triquetral; 6, Barton's fracture.

6 weeks or more until the fracture can be ruled out. **IF** the patient has one or more of the following factors provide support for the wrist and arrange review in the A&E department or the orthopaedic clinic:

- swelling over the anatomical snuff box;
- tenderness in the anatomical snuff box;
- tenderness over the scaphoid tubercule;
- pain on axial compression of the scaphoid;
- patients thought to need scaphoid views (the indication for these views is a clinical suspicion);
- patients with soft-tissue swelling over the dorsum of the wrist on the lateral X-ray.

The treatment of established scaphoid fractures, other carpal bone, radius, and ulnar fractures is well covered in other textbooks. However, a few injuries require special mention:

- *Avulsions from triquetral* — Small fragments are often seen on the dorsum of the wrist on a lateral view. These indicate significant ligamentous injury. Treatment is by a short period of rest then by mobilization.

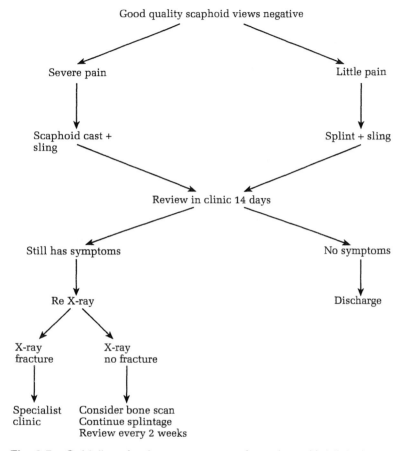

Fig. 8.5 ● Guidelines for the management of a patient with 'clinical scaphoid injury' (Adapted from BAAEM 1992).

- *Hamate fractures* — These are difficult to visualize on X-ray. They may cause ulnar nerve compression. Carpal tunnel views may be required.
- *Carpal dislocations* — These are rare but easily overlooked (see Fig. 8.3) It is important to diagnose these injuries at the time of presentation as neurovascular injury is a common complication. Always check normal carpal alignment.

In children

Epiphyseal fractures, torus (minor compression) fractures, radioulnar fractures, humeral and clavicular fractures
In the younger child accurate localization of the injury may be difficult. The contents list for this section is exclusively of fractures, not a soft-tissue injury in sight! This is because these injuries can be easily overlooked. Always perform a systematic examination or many fractures may be labelled as 'soft-tissue injury' leading to unnecessary pain for the child and much annoyance of the parents.

Take a careful history and examine the whole limb from the clavicle to the hand. Observe the child carefully. Give them a toy to play with and see how the limb is used.

> **A child with a fracture may show no (or minimal) pain on palpation or on full range of movements of the limb**

Older children are more likely to localize their pain, but the difficulty in diagnosis may be in X-ray interpretation. Small torus fractures, undisplaced epiphyseal injuries, and elbow fractures may easily be missed.

If it is impossible to localize the exact site of symptoms in a young child who will not use the limb then the whole limb may need to be X-rayed.

In patients over 50 years of age

Distal radial fractures, radial head fractures, shoulder injury
A fall in the elderly is more likely to cause a fracture or a more severe proximal soft-tissue injury. Distal radial fractures are usually easy to diagnose, but treatment is difficult and the options are outside the scope of this text. The shoulder is prone to develop a traumatic effusion

Trauma — carpal ligament injury

Wrist 'sprains' are complex and controversial subjects where even experienced experts in the field have problems in agreeing the diagnostic criteria and treatment. As with a ligament injury in any other part of the body they present a spectrum of injury from the mild self-limiting Grade 1 injury to complete ruptures of vital supporting ligaments that may cause long-term instability and disability.

The most common ligament injuries in our experience are:

- scapholunate ligament injury;
- triangular cartilage tears/distal radioulnar joint instability;
- dorsiflexed intracalated segment instability (DISI).

Diagnosis may be difficult. These injuries should be suspected where a patient has many symptoms after a fall yet radiographs show no fractures. Careful clinical assessment may indicate the likely diagnosis:

- Pain mainly on the extremes of supination and pain on resisted pronation/supination indicates triangular ligament/radioulnar joint problems.
- Tenderness over the scaphoid with an increased scapholunate gap present.
- DISI is suspected in patients with continuing wrist pain after injury. There may be tenderness over the dorsum of the carpus. A true lateral X-ray with the wrist in neutral shows abnormal carpal alignment with a volar facing lunate and a *Dorsiflexed* capitate (hence the name *Dorsiflexed* intercalated segment instability) and an increased scapholunate angle.

Many other investigations, including further X-rays with varying wrist and hand positions (e.g. a true lateral while gripping), screening of the wrist movements, MRI, or arthroscopy, may be required to make a definitive diagnosis. Most of these will be impossible in many A&E departments, but patients with severe 'wrist sprains' do require follow-up in an appropriate clinic.

Non-trauma — wrist pain? Due to overuse (sofTer)

Paratendinitis crepitans, De Quervain's stenosing tenovaginitis, 'tenosynovitis'

Many patients will present to A&E departments with wrist pain and there may be some suggestion of repetitive activity or overuse. Some may have definite signs of inflammation, but the majority will have none. If there is no swelling, no warmth, no crepitus, no localized specific tenderness, or pain on specific resisted movements then 'tenosynovitis' should not be diagnosed. Such patients are best referred to their GP for full evaluation and specialist referral if necessary.

Paratendinitis crepitans

History

The condition is due to inflammation of the paratendon where the wrist extensors cross the thumb extensors. There is a clear history of activity such as hammering, heavy digging, or brick-laying. There is usually no previous history of upper limb problems. The patient complains of pain and swelling above the wrist. They may say that they can feel the wrist creaking.

Examination

Look — There is significant swelling on the radial side of the wrist in the lower third of the forearm.
Feel — The swollen area is tender and as the wrist is moved there is a characteristic creaking sensation (crepitus).
Move — There is pain on *passive* wrist flexion and especially on ulnar deviation. There is pain on *resisted* wrist extension and resisted thumb extension.

Treatment

This condition almost always settles within 10 days with rest. Immobilization in a scaphoid type plaster or wrist splint is unnecessary, but it does give good pain relief. NSAIDs are used if there are no contraindications.

De Quervain's tenovaginitis

History

This condition is due to thickening of the tendon sheath of long abductor and short extensor tendons to the thumb as they pass over the radial styloid. There is pain on using the wrist and thumb (gripping, lifting). There may be a recent increase is activity (washer-women thumb).

Examination

Look — There may be very subtle swelling over the radial styloid.
Feel — There is specific tenderness over the radial styloid. There may be a palpable lump.
Move — Passive radial deviation of the wrist is very painful. Resisted thumb extension/abduction is painful.

Treatment

Rest is the first-line treatment. Steroid injection and possible surgical decompression may be required if the condition does not settle. The patient is reviewed by their general practitioner.

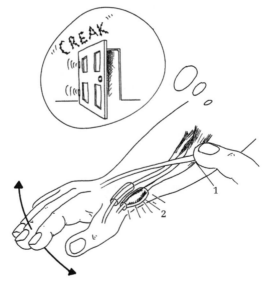

Fig. 8.6 ● Extensor tendon problems. Creaking sensation on wrist flexion and extension of paratendinitis crepitans at the point where the thumb extensors are crossed by the wrist extensors. Stenosing tenovaginitis (De Quervain's) over the radial styloid (pain on radial deviation and resisted thumb abduction).

'Tenosynovitis'

Tenosynovitis indicates inflammation of a specific tendon sheath. It may be caused by infection, rheumatoid disease, and occasionally by overuse. There are very specific signs of swelling over a single tendon, specific tenderness over the tendon with pain on resisted movement and on passive stretch of that tendon. These cases are much less common than the patient who presents saying: 'I have got tenosynovitis'.

History

The pain is often poorly localized and may radiate up and down the limb. There may be a history of a repetitive work task and often there is a history of previous similar episodes.

Examination

Look — There is no swelling. The wrist is often held in a 'limb' fashion with flexion of 45 degrees.
Feel — There is tenderness which is poorly localized and may involve the forearm, wrist, and hand. There is no increased heat.
Move — Most active and passive movements are painful. There is no **specific** resisted movement that reproduces the symptoms.
Nerves — Check the neck and shoulder as referred pain may cause similar presentations. Check the median nerve as carpal tunnel syndrome may cause similar symptoms.

Treatment

The typical case, as described above, should be referred to their GP for further assessment once serious causes of wrist pain have been excluded. If there are no specific signs then do not diagnose 'tenosynovitis' which is a recognized industrial disease; giving this as a diagnosis carries significant medico-legal implications.

Non-trauma — wrist pain and swelling (SOfter tiSsUes)

Septic arthritis, osteoarthritis, rheumatoid arthritis, gout and pseudogout

Presentation — usually elderly patient

History

The patient presents with a sudden pain in the wrist. There is usually a history of previous arthritis. The pain may be severe which keeps the patient awake. Ask about any systemic feature of infection (sweating, feeling hot and cold).

Examination

General — Check the patient's temperature and pulse.
Look — There is significant swelling over both aspects of the wrist and there may be erythema.
Feel — The wrist is warm and very tender.
Move — All movements are very limited by pain.

Investigations

These will depend on the clinical assessment. While an acute on chronic inflammatory condition (psuedogout, osteo/ rheumatoid arthritis) is the most likely cause, the signs and symptoms are very similar to septic arthrits. X-ray may show calcification within the joint and the triangular cartilage. The ESR and white-blood count should be checked as should plasma urate levels. Joint aspiration should be considered.

Treatment

If the patient is pyrexial, has systemic symptoms, or the ESR and white count are raised then the patient is referred to the orthopaedic team to rule out septic arthritis. If the patient is well and inflammatory conditions seem the most likely cause, advise rest, and a non-steroidal anti-inflammatory agent (**caution** with NSAIDs in the elderly — use a short course, moderate dose). The patient should be reviewed within 24–48 hours. In most acute on chronic conditions the symptoms will have subsided. Continuing severe symptoms require referral.

Presentation — wrist pain and swelling in younger person

Ganglion, missed fractures, Keinbock's disease

Ganglion — is a localized out-pouching of the synovial lining of a joint or tendon sheath. It may occur acutely after trauma or arise spontaneously. There is a characteristic localized swelling with no other symptoms. It is usually not tender. The patient may be referred to their GP for further follow-up and appropriate referral.

Missed fractures — In the younger patient significant swelling of the wrist joint proper should be fully investigated. Missed fractures, especially of the scaphoid still occur.

Keinbock's disease — is an osteochondritis of the lunate. As with missed fractures the diagnosis can only be made on X-ray.

Carpal instability — should be considered (see above).

Wrist and hand pain, no swelling

Diagnoses to consider include carpal tunnel syndrome and ulnar nerve compression (see Chapter 9).

Pitfalls and how to avoid them

- *Missed fracture of the scaphoid.* This is one of the commonest causes for complaint and litigation. The difficulty in diagnosing this injury has been widely known for many years yet cases are still missed. Experienced A&E doctors will be unhappy to diagnose a 'wrist sprain' on a single visit in a young person with a typical history.
- *Missing fractures in a child.* These may be difficult to diagnose. After a full examination and X-ray if a child is not using a limb then either ask someone more senior (Box 8.1)

to see the child or tell the parents that the cause of the pain is not obvious. Rest the limb in a sling or collar and cuff and bring the child back for review by a senior in 1–2 days.

- *Carpal dislocations.* The history is of significant trauma and the wrist is very swollen and painful. The X-ray appearances are diagnostic but often missed. Ensure the 'three Cs are in alignment' (Fig. 8.3).

Box 8.1 • What would a senior do?

- Take a full history with details of the mechanism of injury.
- Take a full previous history.
- Chat to the parents and child to establish rapport.
- Watch the child play, and play with the child.
- Examine the **normal** limb.
- Examine the limb commencing at the sternoclavicular joint.
- Note **any** reaction to specific palpation/movement however slight.
- Possibly X-ray the whole limb, including the clavicle.
- Advise patients that there is no obvious serious injury but it can be difficult to exclude a more minor injury.
- Offer support, analgesia, and early review (1–3 days)
- Advise parents that they may return if symptoms increase or new symptoms develop.
- Give phone number where they may book an early clinic return visit.

Further reading

1. Barton, N. (1989). Repetitive strain disorder — often misdiagnosed and often not work related. *British Medical Journal,* **299,** 405–6.
2. British Association of Accident and Emergency Medicine. (1992). The management of suspected scaphoid fracture. London.
3. Chidgey, L. K. (1992). Chronic wrist pain. *Orthopedic Clinics of North America,* **23,** 49–64.
4. DaCruz, D. and Dias, J. (1990). Traumatic wrist pain. *Hospital Update,* 665–657.

5. Green, D. P. (1993). Carpal dislocations and instabilities. In *Operative hand surgery* (ed. D. P. Green), pp. 881–919. Churchill Livingstone, New York.
6. Lamb, D. W., Hooper, G., and Kuczynski, K. (1989). *The practise of hand surgery* (2nd edn). Blackwell Scientific, Edinburgh
7. Thurson, E. and Szabo, R. M. (1992). Common tendinitis problems in the hand and forearm. *Orthopedic Clinics of North America*, **23**, 65–73.

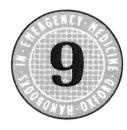

The hand

Key points

* Anatomy
  — The hand is a highly complex structure capable of tasks as diverse as power grip, punching, and high speed, delicate, precise actions.
  — It is also a highly sensitive sense organ.
  — Minor injury can lead to permanent disability either in work or leisure pastimes.
  — Joints depend on ligaments for stability.
  — Complete tears can lead to an unstable joint,
* Trauma
  — Exclude bony injury by X-ray.
  — Exclude rotational deformity.
  — Never dismiss ligament injury (or small bony avulsions from the insertions of ligaments) as trivial injuries. Even a Grade 2 sprain of a PIPJ will take 3 months to recover.
  — Test joint stability.
  — Tendon ruptures are common yet easily missed.
  — Treat possible Boutonnière injury on suspicion.
* Non-trauma
  — Deep abscesses cause severe pain yet fluctuation may not be evident.
  — Tendon sheath infections cause severe pain on passive stretch.
  — Osteomyelitis of the terminal phalanx is common.
  — Gout is common but may be difficult to differentiate from septic arthritis.

Anatomy

Terminology

Use names of fingers rather than numbers. Describe the borders of the hand/fingers as **radial** and **ulnar** (see Fig. 9.1). Use palmar and dorsal to describe the surfaces of the hand and fingers rather than front and back.

Joints

The **joints** all follow the same basic pattern (see Fig. 9.2) The capsule is very strong over the anterior aspect where it is

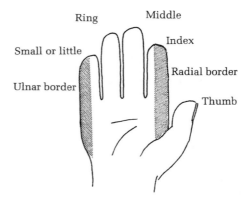

Fig. 9.1 ● Name fingers and use the terms 'ulnar' and 'radial' to describe the borders of the hand/fingers.

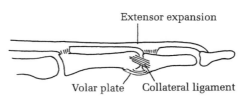

Fig. 9.2 ● PIPJ. The volar plate, collateral ligaments, and the extensor expansion are the main stabilizing structures.

specialized into a **volar plate**. This structure resists hyper-extension stress and is often damaged in the common injury 'bent finger back'. The collateral ligaments (radial and ulnar) resist lateral forces. Rupture of these ligaments may cause significant disability as can rupture of the ulnar collateral ligament of the thumb metacarpophalangeal joint.

Movements

The movements of the fingers are performed by four major muscle groups:

- **Extrinsic flexors** (flexors profundus and superficialis, pollicis longus);
- **Extrinsic extensors** (extensors digitorum, indicis, digiti minimi, pollicis longus);
- **Intrinsic flexors** (interossei and lumbricals flex the metacarpophalangeal joints)
- **Intrinsic extensors** (interossei and lumbricals extend the interphalangeal joints)

Finger movements and hand function are a complex balance between these groups of muscles. Their actions are summarized in Figs 9.3A–D. The extrinsic flexors act at the interphalangeal joints while the intrinsic muscles flex the metacarpophalangeal joints. Conversely, the extrinsic extensors act mainly at the metacarpophalangeal joint and the intrinsic muscles extend the interphalangeal joints

Examination

Joint above — Examine the wrist.
Look — Note the exact position of swelling bruising. Often this is generalized around a joint but may be much more localized (e.g. over one of the collateral ligaments). Comparison with the normal hand/digit is essential. *Lateral and antero-posterior deformity* of the fingers is usually easily seen but *rotational deformity* is less obvious. Look at the fingers 'end on' and note the orientation of the nails (Fig. 9.4A). Also ask the patient to gently flex the fingers, this will make such a deformity much more obvious (Fig. 9.4B).

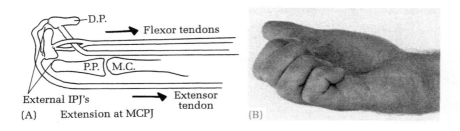

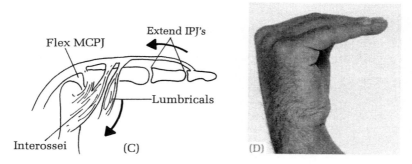

Fig. 9.3 ● Function of the extrinsic muscles (A,B). The extrinsics flex the IPJs and extend the MCPJ. The intrinsic muscles flex the MCPJ and extend the IPJ (C,D).

Table 9.1 ● Abbreviations used

Joints		Tendons	
CMCJ:	carpometacarpal joint	ABL:	abductor pollicis longus
DIPJ:	distal interphalangeal joint	EPL:	extensor pollicis longus
IPJ:	interphalangeal (thumb) joint	Ext Dig:	extensor digitorum
MCPJ:	metacarpophalangeal joint	FPL:	flexor pollicis longus
PIPJ:	proximal interphalangeal joint	FDP:	flexor digitorum profundus
		FDS:	flexor digitorum superficialis

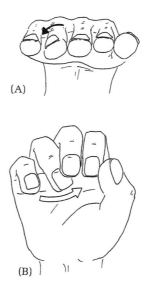

Fig. 9.4 ● Rotation deformity of fingers. Look at the nails 'end on' (A). If a rotational deformity is present then the nail plate will not lie in the same plane. The deformity is much more obvious on flexion of the fingers (B).

Feel — Accurate gentle palpation aims to localize the exact points of maximum tenderness.

Move — Active and passive ranges of joint motion are noted. Stress the collateral ligament of the joint involved or Grade 3 injuries will be missed (see p 000).

Test tendon function. An initial screening test is to ask the patient to make a fist and then to fully extend the fingers. Then the relevant tests are carried out, testing specific tendons:

FDP is tested by checking the range of flexion at the DIPJ. Take care to isolate the DIPJ as flexion of the PIPJ can cause *apparent* DIPJ flexion. Also test resisted flexion.

FDS is the main flexor of the PIPJ, but to specifically test this muscle the FDP must be inactivated. This is achieved by holding the other fingers fully extended (this fully stretches

FDP which has a *single* muscle belly). The patient is then asked to flex the PIPJ, confirming that the FDS is intact (Figs 9.5 A,B). *Extensor communis* is simple to test by asking the patient to fully extend the MCPJ. If any tendon is not functioning then the finger will 'drop'. Note that it is still possible to extend the PIPJ and the DIPJ due to the action of the intrinsic muscles (Fig. 9.6). *The extensor mechanism* over the PIPJ is complex. It divides into three parts. The middle slip inserts into the base of the

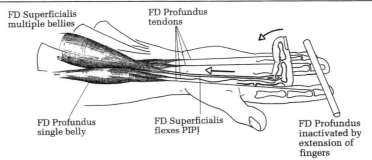

FD Superficialis multiple bellies

FD Profundus tendons

FD Profundus single belly

FD Superficialis flexes PIPJ

FD Profundus inactivated by extension of fingers

(A)

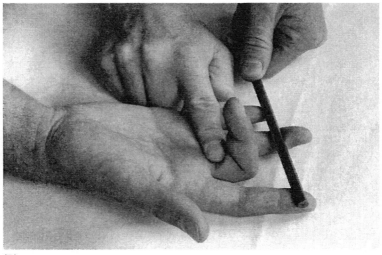

(B)

Fig. 9.5 • (A,B), FDS testing. Hold the other fingers straight to disable the FDP. Check flexion of the PIPJ.

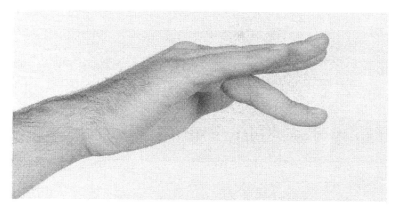

Fig. 9.6 ● Extensor communis. Ask the patient to extend the MCPJ.

middle phalanx and is responsible for extending the PIPJ **and** it is the main stabilizer of the PIPJ dorsally. It is difficult to test in isolation. The best way to do this is to flex the finger over a flat surface (tabletop) and then to ask the patient to

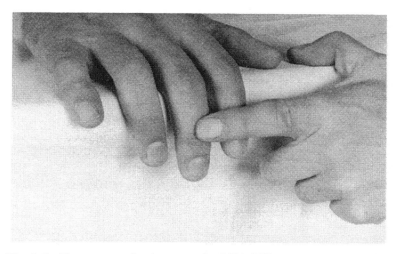

Fig. 9.7 ● Extensor mechanism over the PIPJ. Difficult to test in isolation. Weakness and pain on resisted extension may indicate middle slip rupture.

extend the finger against resistance. **Note** any weakness might indicate a middle slip injury. (**NB** the patient will still be able to extend the joint initially — see Boutonnière deformity p. 165 Fig. 9.12.)

The extensor of the DIPJ is easily tested by checking active and resisted extension over the DIPJ.

Trauma — bent thumb back/out

Assessment and treatment

History

This is of a hyperextension injury to the thumb or an abduction injury (e.g. common skiing injury).

Examination

Look — There is swelling and bruising around the joint(s) involved. The MCPJ is most commonly involved in ligamentous injury. The same mechanism may cause fractures around the CMCJ (e.g. Bennet's) or of the terminal phalanx (often complex involving the joint).

Feel — Try to pinpoint the exact points of maximum tenderness. For example, which is the most tender: the radial collateral ligament, the ulnar collateral ligament, the volar capsule, or the dorsal capsule?

Move — Active and passive movements will be restricted. Assess joint stability (with the joint flexed to 20–30 degrees). Seek evidence of ulnar collateral ligament instability (Figs 9.8A,B). Local anaesthetic may make this test easier to perform.

Investigations

X-ray — Small avulsions from the base of the proximal phalanx/head of the metacarpal are significant and indicate ligamentous avulsion. If the injury is to the CMCJ then examine closely for a Bennett's-type fracture/dislocation. Injuries to the IPJ are often severe and may involve subluxation (Fig. 9.9.)

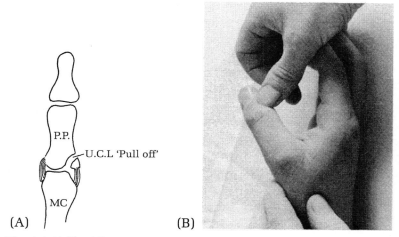

Fig. 9.8 (A,B) • Ulnar collateral ligament instability. Test with the MCPJ flexed to 30 degrees.

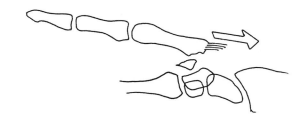

Fig. 9.9 • Bennett's fracture dislocation. Muscles pull the thumb metacarpal proximally, the small fracture fragment remains in the correct position.

Treatment

Sprains of the MCPJ need careful assessment. If there is evidence of instability seek advice. Surgical repair of the ulnar collateral ligament is sometimes required. This injury is very painful and causes significant disability. Moderate injury (Grade 2 sprain) may require a Plaster of Paris thumb spica for

10 days. Less severe injuries are given a support (a rigid thumb spica) and advised that the injury will take some months to settle. Patients in manual occupations may require occupational therapy.

Trauma — bent finger back

Assessment and treatment

The main structure preventing hyperextension is the volar plate (see Fig. 9.2). This may be torn or the attachment of this ligament to the base of the middle phalanx may be fractured (see Fig. 9.13). This is a very common injury and one that causes significant disability, the average case may take 2–3 months to settle.

History

Generally, this is of a hyperextension injury, but note if there has been lateral stress in addition as this might indicate that a collateral ligament may have been damaged. The patient's occupation and leisure pastimes may indicate a need for more active treatment (e.g. musician).

Examination

Look and feel — to pinpoint the exact points of maximum tenderness. Specifically, check if one or both of the collateral ligaments are the site of swelling or tenderness.
Move — Active and passive range will be reduced. Test for stability of the collateral ligaments by applying gentle lateral force with the finger flexed to 30–40 degrees (delay until after X-ray). Check tendon function.

Investigations

X-ray — Always X-ray these injuries and look for small avulsion fractures from the base of the middle phalanx or from the attachments of the collateral ligaments. Also check that there is no evidence of subluxation.

Treatment

Minor Grade 1 and 2 injuries of **one** ligament can be treated with simple support by strapping the injured finger to its neighbour for 7–10 days. Advise the patient that the injury may take some months to settle. If the patient has high functional demands on the fingers consider specialist referral. More severe injuries, fractures, Grade 3 tears of one or more ligaments require follow-up in an appropriate clinic. Such injuries are best treated initially with a rigid splint that limits extension but allows flexion (extension block splint).

Trauma — hit on end of finger

A direct forceful blow to the end of the extended finger often causes significant injury. The force may be transmitted along the finger causing ligament and/or bony damage to any of the finger joints. Locate the exact area of maximum tenderness and check stability. Obtain X-rays and exclude intra-articular fractures or subluxations.

Trauma — 'hit a wall' (punch injury)

Assessment and treatment

The patient may not be telling the whole truth regarding this mechanism of injury! Punch-type injuries are very common and often cause significant structural damage.

Examination

Look — Note the exact sites of swelling and check for deformity, especially rotational deformity (Fig. 9.4). Any wounds over the MCPJ may well signify a tooth injury that may have penetrated the MCPJ.
Feel — Note the exact sites of tenderness.
Move — Check the stability of the joints and tendon function, especially extensor tendon function over the MCPJ and PIPJ (see Fig 9.6, 9.7).

Investigations

X-ray — Obtain the correct views (e.g. hand **or** finger). If there is marked tenderness around the base of the little finger and ring finger metacarpals and the CMCJ, ask for a *true lateral of the hand*. Dislocations of the CMCJ often involve fractures of the metacarpal bases and are often unstable injuries (Fig. 9.10).

> **Dislocations of the CMCJ are easily missed — take true lateral view of the hand**

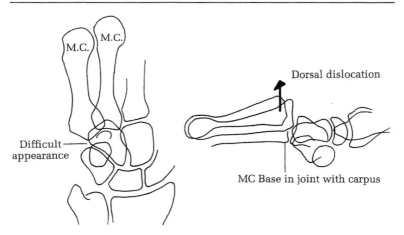

Fig. 9.10 • Carpometacarpal joint dislocation. Easily missed. Suspect with local tenderness over the base of the little/ring finger metacarpals and get a true lateral X-ray of the hand.

Treatment

Fractures of the little finger metacarpal neck are managed according to departmental guidelines, but often simple neighbour strapping is all that is required.

Wounds over the little finger MCPJ should be explored to exclude tendon damage and joint penetration. These injuries always require antibiotics and follow-up.

Dislocations of the CMCJ need referral to the orthopaedic team. *Direct blows* to the dorsum of the PIPJ need careful assessment and follow-up to prevent Boutonnière deformity.

Trauma — dislocated finger

The common dislocations are to the interphalangeal joints. These are usually easily diagnosed and often the patient has reduced the dislocation themselves. X-rays should be taken to exclude fractures. Following reduction an assessment is made of ligament stability. Postreduction X-rays are taken to ensure complete relocation of the joint.

Simple dislocations may be treated by neighbour strapping and review is advised in 5–7 days.

Incomplete reduction, gross instability, or significant intra-articular fractures should be referred to the hand surgeons.

Dislocations of the MCPJ are less common. The diagnosis is obvious. However, some of these injuries are irreducible as the base of the phalanx will have buttonholed through the joint capsule or the volar plate may be stuck in the joint. If you have problems in reducing this injury refer to the hand surgeons. Reduction is attempted by flexing the wrist then pushing the proximal phalanx back into place. Obtain a check X-ray and splint the finger with flexion at the MCPJ.

Trauma — finger will not bend/straighten (closed tendon ruptures)

This may occur after trauma, usually due to fractures or tendon rupture, or it may occur in the absence of trauma (see Trigger finger/thumb, locked MCPJ). Tendon ruptures, both traumatic and spontaneous will be discussed in this section.

Apparent inability to move or straighten a finger may be due to displaced fracture or major joint injury

---

Flexor digitorum profundus

History

This is of a forced extension against a forceable contraction of the muscle (e.g. a climber 'hanging on by his fingers' slips or a hand gripping a rugby jersey is pulled away).

Examination

Look — There is swelling around the DIPJ.
Feel — There is tenderness over the volar aspect of the DIPJ and tendon sheath.
Move — There is no active flexion at the DIPJ (passive flexion is relatively pain-free.)

Treatment

Refer these injuries for surgical repair.

Extensor tendon over DIPJ 'Mallet finger'

History

After an episode of relatively minor trauma the patient is unable to extend the DIPJ.

Examination

Look — There is an obvious 'mallet' deformity.
Feel — There is tenderness over the base of the distal phalanx.
Move — Active extension is absent. Passive extension is relatively pain-free.

Investigations

X-ray — Often there is a small fragment of bone avulsed from the base of the distal phalanx. Check that there is no volar subluxation.

Treatment

If there is no fracture or the fracture fragment is small (less than one-third of the joint surface) then treat in a mallet finger

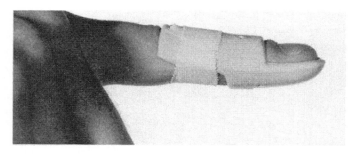

Fig. 9.11 ● Mallet finger splint. Give the patient advice on its correct use.

extension splint (Fig. 9.11). The splint is worn for 8 weeks. The patient is advised that they may remove the splint to wash the finger but when they do so the finger **must** be kept straight (e.g. by keeping the finger on a flat surface). After washing, the finger is carefully dried and the splint replaced.

If there is a large fracture fragment then seek further advice, surgery may be required especially if there is subluxation at the joint.

Blow to the dorsum of the PIPJ — injury to the central slip of the extensor tendon

> **This is a difficult diagnosis which can result in loss of the finger if missed — treat on suspicion**

Anatomy

The extensor expansion divides into three slips: the central slip and two lateral bands. If the central slip is divided then extension is still possible at the PIPJ due to the intact lateral bands. However, over a period of a few weeks repeated normal flexion of the finger results in the gradual migration of the lateral bands to the sides of the finger. The result is a 'button-holing' (Boutonnière deformity) through the tendon with a resultant fixed-flexion deformity at the PIPJ and a hyperexten-sion deformity at the DIPJ, (Fig. 9.12).

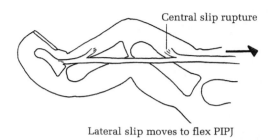

Central slip rupture

Lateral slip moves to flex PIPJ

Fig. 9.12 • Boutonièrre deformity. Rupture of the central slip of the extensor expansion allows the head of the metacarpal to buttonhole through the lateral slips.

History

There is a history of a significant blow with some force to the dorsum of the PIPJ (e.g. a spanner slipping and the motor mechanic striking his knuckle on the edge of the engine).

Examination

Look — There is very localized swelling and bruising over the dorsum of the PIPJ.
Feel — There is specific tenderness over the joint line.
Move — **Extension at the joint is intact** (immediately after the injury). Place the finger over the edge of a table and test resisted extension. This may be weak and painful.

Investigation

X-ray — Normal.

Treatment

With a good history and specific localized signs this injury needs to be treated on suspicion. The finger is splinted in extension (using a Zimmer splint) and the patient brought back for review to a clinic in 1 week. Usually the joint is kept extended for 3 weeks then mobilized in a dynamic extension splint (Capner splint).

Other tendon ruptures

These usually occur in the presence of other pathology. Extensor pollicis longus tendon may rupture in the months after a Colles' fracture. Other tendons may rupture in rheumatoid arthritis. Refer such injuries for repair or tendon transfer.

Trauma — crushed hand/finger

This is a common presentation, especially to the distal phalanx area. The topic is discussed more fully in another book in this series (see *wounds and burns book*). These injuries should be X-rayed. Treatment is primarily aimed at re-aligning the soft tissues, replacing the nail if it is out of the nail bed, and releasing subungual haematomas. Antibiotics are given if there is a fracture and the patient advised to keep the limb elevated (sitting with elbow on cushion and hand raised).

Compartment syndrome can occur in the small muscles of the hand and any patient with very severe pain after a crush injury should be referred to the hand surgeons for a further opinion.

Non-trauma — pain and swelling in hand/finger

Sepsis, osteoarthritis, fractures missed/pathological, seropositive arthritis, gout

Sepsis (Softer)

Paronychia, pulp. space infection, herpetic whitlow, osteomyelitis, septic arthritis, tendon sheath infection, cellulitis, and lymphangitis
The hand is perhaps the commonest site for severe soft-tissue infection. Although most infections are easily treated as an outpatient an early review (by the GP or in clinic) is advised as limb-or even life-threatening complications may occur.

History

The main complaint is of pain, often throbbing in nature. Severe pain indicates an abscess or tendon sheath infection. Ask if there is any history of a penetrating injury (splinter or bite). In patients with pre-existing arthritis, sepsis is still a possible cause of an acute arthritis.

Beware of a prolonged history of pain and swelling, especially in the pulp, this often indicates osteomyelitis.

Examination

This should include the temperature and pulse rate and checking the epitrochlear (just proximal to the medial epicondyle of the elbow) and axillary lymph nodes.

Look — There is swelling of the affected area. Note any wounds or healing scars. In deep infections there is marked swelling on the *dorsum* of the hand. Look for spreading cellulitis or ascending lymphangitis.

Feel — The area is hot and tender. Fluctuation may be present.

Move *Septic arthritis* — all movements of the joint are very painful.

Tendon sheath infection — extreme pain on passive stretch of the tendon or on resisted movement.

Investigations

X-ray — Indicated if a foreign body is suspected or if there is a possibility of osteomyelitis.

Treatment

Superficial localized (paronychia, pulp space abscess, furuncle on dorsum of PIPJ) — Incise and drain, give antibiotics if spreading cellulitis.

Superficial spreading (cellulitis, lymphangitis) — If the patient is not toxic give an intramuscular dose of penicillin and co-amoxiclav (Augmentin) or flucloxicillin. Oral antibiotics are prescribed and the patient advised to return if the symptoms become worse, especially if systemic symptoms occur. Review by the GP the following day is advised.

Deep abscess in palm or finger, suspected *osteomyelitis septic arthritis tendon sheath infection* — Refer to hand surgeons/ orthopaedics.

Osteoarthritis (sOfter)

Many patients will have signs of osteoarthritis in the hands, but few will present to A & E. Osteoarthritis of the trape-sometacarpal joint at the base of the thumb may present problems in managing the older patient who has fallen onto an outstretched hand. The joint is very near the scaphoid, and tenderness over and pain on moving the joint may mimic signs of a 'clinical scaphoid' (see p 000). It may be necessary to follow the 'scaphoid routine' for 2 weeks, but after this time accurate localization of the problem is usually possible and after 2 sets of radiographs it is usually safe to mobilize the hand.

Acute swelling in a previously arthritic joint should be assessed with great care. Septic arthritis is rare but is more common in such abnormal joints.

Fractures missed, pathological (soFter)

Small avulsion fractures are frequently overlooked as are the major ligament injuries that may be indicated by such fractures. Patients with localized joint swelling should be X-rayed.

Endochondromas are common and may give rise to pathological fractures.

Seropositive arthritis (tiSsues)

Rheumatoid hand problems might take a whole book to describe, but it is unusual for such patients to present to an A&E department unless there is a sudden change in their condition. *Septic arthritis* should be suspected in a patient with a sudden acute arthritis only affecting a single joint. Tendon ruptures, joint subluxations, or locking of a joint may require referral.

Gout (Urate (tissUes)

Gout may cause acute arthritis in the small joint of the hand but extra-articular depositions of urate (*tophi*) can become acutely inflamed. The appearances may be confused with an acute abscess (commonest over the DIPJ where they might be diagnosed as a paronychia). These episodes may resolve with treatment with a non-steroidal anti-inflammatory agent, but occasionally incision and drainage may be required.

Non-trauma — sticking and clicking fingers/thumb

T, tendon problems

Trigger finger/thumb, paediatric trigger thumb
These conditions are caused by thickening of the flexor tendon and/or the sheath at the point where the tendon enters the synovial sheath at the level of the MCPJ.

The condition may be congenital (although it may present later when the inability to flex the digit is noticed by parents).

Other causes of loss of movement include closed tendon ruptures, and occasionally loose bodies in the MCPJ may caused locking of that joint.

History

The patient presents with either clicking in the digit or with an inability to move the digit. There is no history of trauma. In trigger finger/thumb the symptoms are often worse in the morning.

Examination

There is a tender nodule over the tendon at the level of the MCPJ. As the patient flexes the digit a clicking sensation is felt.

Treatment

A typical case responds well to steroid injection into the tendon sheath (*not the tendon*, see Chapter 5). Infants with the condition should be referred to the orthopaedic team.

Non-trauma — pain in hand, no swelling

Referred pain and neural compression, ischaemia

Referred pain and neurological compression (softeR)

Carpal tunnel syndrome is one of the most common peripheral neural entrapment syndromes.

The compression is usually at the level of the wrist in the
carpal tunnel, but it may be at the elbow (as the nerve runs
through pronator teres) or even above the elbow. Occasionally
the anterior interosseous nerve (the main motor branch of the
median nerve in the forearm) may be compressed resulting in
weakness but no sensory symptoms.

History

The patient complains of pain and paraesthesia in the hand,
usually limited to the distribution of the median nerve. The pain
is often worse at night and relieved by elevation. There may be a
history of recent trauma, pregnancy, or thyroid problems.

Examination

There is usually no swelling. Wasting of the thenar muscles is
a late sign. Palpation or percussion over the nerve may cause
the pain and paraesthesia.

Movements are checked, especially the strength of opposi-
tion and thumb abduction. Also check the function of FPL and
the finger flexors. Sensation is examined in detail. Ask the
patient to flex the wrist and to remain in this position for
1 minute. This may provoke the patient's symptoms.

Treatment

The diagnosis must be suspected on the basis of the characteristic history. Most cases can be referred to the GP for further
referral and treatment, but urgent referral to orthopaedics is
required for:

• severe and progressive symptoms;

- evidence of wasting;
- sensory loss.

The ulnar nerve may be compressed at the elbow or the wrist. The sensory symptoms involve the ring and small finger and the motor weakness of the intrinsic hand muscles (the ulnar part of FDP if the compression is at the elbow).

Ischaemia, vascular imbalance (tIssues)

Raynaud's phenomenon is common but patients seldom present to A&E.
Sudek's atrophy is a problem that can be encountered after an injury, especially if there has been a period of Plaster of Paris immobilization. The hand is warm, with shiny erythematous skin, swelling, and pain. Such patients should be referred for an orthopaedic opinion.
Embolic episodes may rarely cause localized subcutaneous bruising to develop, check the blood pressure in both arms. Palpate both radial pulses while elevating the arms above the shoulders and exercising the hands while depressing the shoulders. Listen for cardiac murmurs and subclavian murmurs. Refer these patients for a vascular opinion.

Non-trauma — weakness in hand

Nerve palsy, thoracic outlet compression, cervical radiculopathy, peripheral neuropathy

Nerve palsy

Median and ulnar nerve palsy are discussed above.
Radial nerve palsy resulting in a dropped wrist is common with characteristic weakness of the wrist extensors/and MCPJ extension. The typical history is of prolonged external pressure over the nerve (e.g. 'Saturday night palsy' or 'Crutch palsy'). The patient is given a splint that keeps the wrist and fingers extended and referred for follow-up. Recovery usually takes 6–10 weeks.

Table 9.2 • Compression signs

Structure	Sensory signs	Motor signs
C6	Front/radial side forearm/wrist	Biceps, brachioradialis
C7	Back/radial forearm; index, middle, ring fingers	Triceps, wrist
C8	Ulnar forearm; ring, small finger	Thumb extensors, finger extensors
T1	Inner arm/forearm	Intrinsic hand muscles

Cervical nerve roots or the brachial plexus

These can be compressed or irritated by degenerative osteo-phytes, prolapsed intervertebral discs, cervical ribs, or apical lung tumours. The signs and symptoms will depend on the nerve root involved. (Table 9.2). Some patients with rapidly progressive neurological signs will require urgent referral (mandatory if there are any *lower* limb symptoms or signs).

Other compression syndromes that may affect hand and wrist function include the *anterior interosseous nerve* (weakness of FPL and FDP to index and middle fingers), *the posterior interosseous nerve* (thumb abduction).

Peripheral neuropathy

This may occasionally present with weakness of the hand (often ulnar nerve). Alcohol and diabetes are the commonest causes in A&E practice.

Pitfalls and how to avoid them

- *Missed fractures.* The hand is so vital to everyday function that accurate diagnosis is essential.
- *Take the correct views.* If the injury is to the finger ask for finger views (true lateral and anteroposterior). The oblique view used for the hand does not show the PIPJ and DIPJ well enough to exclude significant fractures.

- If the injury is to the **base** of the metacarpal ask for an additional true lateral view of the hand in addition to the normal AP and oblique views. Fractures and dislocations of the MC–CJ are often missed. The addition of the lateral view helps this diagnosis (the same as for metatarsotarsal joint injury in the foot — see Lisfranc fractures.)
- Commonly missed injuries are summarized in Fig. 9.13.
- *Incorrect splintage.* Rest is important in the early stages of hand injury. If the hand is to be splinted then this should be in the 'position of function' (see Fig. 9.3D). The MCPJ is flexed and the IPJ's extended.
- *Incorrect/insufficient elevation.* The proper way to elevate the limb has been discussed previously (see Fig. 2.1). It is important to explain this to patients stressing that this is an essential part of the treatment.
- *Underestimation of effects of injury.* The inexperienced are likely to give very optimistic prognoses for hand injury. Even a relatively minor injury (e.g. 'bent finger back') will often result in significant disability for 3 months. The patient should be advised that the injury will take some time to resolve. Review should be arranged for significant joint injuries where there are signs of instability or any fracture (even the smallest avulsion indicates severe ligament injury), especially if the patient has high functional demands.

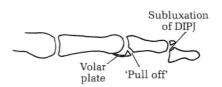

Fig. 9.13 ● Missed fractures. Always get a true lateral of the finger. Check for small intra-articular fractures, especially at the insertion of the volar plate.

Further reading

1. Atasoy, E. (1996). Thoracic outlet compression syndrome. *Orthopedic Clinics of North America*, **27**, 265–303.
2. Bowers, W. H. (1987). *The interphalangeal joints*. Churchill Livingstone, Edinburgh.
3. Dray, G. J. and Eason, R. G. (1993). Dislocations and ligament injuries in the digits. In *Operative hand surgery* (ed. D. P. Green), 787–191. Churchill Livingstone, New York.
4. Lamb, D. W., Hooper, G., and Kuczynski, K. (1989). *The practise of hand surgery* (2nd edn). Blackwell Scientific, Edinburgh.
5. Neviaser, R. J. (1993). Dislocations and ligament injuries of the digits. In *Operative orthopaedics*, (2nd edn). (ed. M. W. Chapman), pp. 1237–50. J. B. Lippincott, Philadelphia.
6. Newland, C. C. (1992). Gamekeeper's thumb. *Orthopedic Clinics of North America*, **27**, 265–303.

Hip and thigh

Key points

- Trauma — Falls in patients over 50 years of age
  — Hip fractures are common — always X-ray patients.
  — Fractures may not be visible on initial films, admission/
  follow-up, bone scan may be required.
  — Elderly patients, living alone, rendered immobile by a
  fall may require admission or nursing-home care.
- Trauma — Direct blow to the thigh
  — May cause large intramuscular haematoma.
  — Refer if patient unable to flex knee beyond 90 degrees.
  — May go on to develop myosotis ossificans.
- Trauma — Injury to quadriceps/patellar tendon
  — Often missed.
  — Minor injury or stumble in elderly.
  — Always test straight-leg raising.
  — Refer patient if unable to straight-leg raise.
- Non-trauma — Limping child
  — Diagnoses include: septic arthritis; missed fractures
  (tibia); Perthes disease; **slipped upper femoral epi-
  physis**, referred abdo/back pain; osteosarcoma; juvenile
  rheumatoid diseases; 'irritable hip'; Henoch–Schönlien
  purpura.
  — This presentation needs a very full history, examination,
  and investigation. If admission is not required, careful
  early follow-up is advised.

Anatomy and function

The hip is a classical 'ball and socket' joint, surrounded by large muscle groups that allow the stable transmission of bodyweight with every running or walking stride.

The major movements of the hip are outlined in Fig. 10.1.

The femur provides the bony skeleton for the thigh and is almost completely covered by bulky muscle groups such as quadriceps, and the hamstrings (biceps femoris, semimembranosis, and semitendinosis).

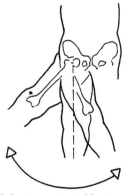

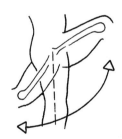

Flexion 110° : Extension 30°

Abduction 50° : Adduction 30°

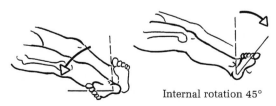

Internal rotation 45°

External rotation 45°

Fig. 10.1 • Range of hip movements.

Examination

The patient should be undressed.

Joint above — Examine the back and abdomen in difficult cases or where there is no clear history of trauma. Aortic rupture, acute abdomen, and spinal cord/cauda equina compression may all present as hip pain.

Look — Observe any deformity or swelling. If the hip is held in flexion this is highly suggestive of a joint effusion. A shortened externally rotated leg is suggestive of a fracture of the neck of femur. **Note:** if the leg appears to be shorter than the other ensure that the pelvis is level.

Feel — The hip joint is deep, but other structures such as the pubic superior pubic ramus can be palpated as can many of the muscles and tendons such as quadriceps and the adductors. Specific tenderness over the greater trochanter may indicate a bursitis.

Move — Commence by moving the opposite hip (see Thomas' test below Fig. 10.2). Passive range includes comparison of flexion/extension/adduction/abduction and the rotations. The characteristic reduction of movement (*capsular pattern*) is that of a hip held in at 30 degrees and limitation of rotation, especially internal rotation.

Function — Always try to observe the patient standing and walking. This may reveal a pelvic tilt or an abnormal gait.

Nerves and vessels — Exclude any neural deficit that may arise from a back problem. Examine the aorta and major limb pulses.

Trauma — hip pain after a fall (the elderly)

This is a common and ever-expanding problem and over half these patients will have significant pathology, often a fractured neck of the femur or a fracture of the pelvis.

Careful history and assessment are obtained and X-rays taken of the affected hip and pelvis. Even if the X-rays are normal and the patient has pain on weight bearing, then there still may be a fracture.

In this group it may be impossible to discharge the patient home if they cannot weight bear and they live alone. Such patients warrant careful consideration. Local guidelines should indicate the management of these patients and who is responsible for this assessment and continuing care. If the patient can be discharged then they should be brought back for review in 4–5 days time to ensure that symptoms are settling. If weight bearing is still difficult then further X-rays or a bone scan are indicated.

Trauma — direct/indirect to thigh

Quadriceps haematoma, muscle tear, quadriceps rupture

Direct blow

History

This is a common sporting injury especially in rugby and football. The player is struck over the quadriceps area by an opponent. There is localized tenderness with swelling over the muscle.

Examination

Examination shows normal hip movements but knee movements are restricted, especially in flexion. There is not normally a knee effusion in the early stages of this condition, but a reactive effusion may develop after 2 days. *Test straight-leg raising to* ensure extensor mechanism integrity.

Treatment

Treatment is symptomatic with the application of local measures, rest, elevation, and cessation of sporting activities. If the knee cannot be bent past 90 degrees of flexion then this indicates a severe haematoma and complete rest is advised. Crutches are given. Stretching of the muscle is contraindicated at this stage and the patient is followed-up regularly in the A&E clinic or by the orthopaedic team. The complication of myositis ossificans may follow this injury.

Sudden pain in the thigh after a definite history of injury

Muscle belly tear/quadriceps tendon rupture/partial tendon rupture
Tears of part of the quadriceps muscle are common. Tears and strains of the hamstrings are common. The most severe injury is a complete tear of the quadriceps tendon as it inserts into the patella. The patient is usually elderly and gives a history of severe pain, just above the knee after stumbling. The patient cannot weight bear.

Straight-leg raising must be tested or this clinical diagnosis will be overlooked

---

Minor tears of biceps femoris are common in athletes. Sometimes there is an avulsion fracture from the anterior superior iliac spine. Complete tears of the quadriceps muscle and certainly tears of the quadriceps tendon require surgical repair. More minor tears of part of the quadriceps or hamstrings are treated symptomatically.

Non-trauma — limping child

A child may present with a limp or with pain in the hip or knee or leg. There may be no history of trauma or only minimal trauma.

Differential diagnoses in this common presentation include (see also Table 10.1):

- septic arthritis (any patient);
- reactive arthritis (irritable hip), 2–6 years;
- Perthes' disease, 5–8 years;
- slipped epiphysis, 9–16 years;
- congenital dislocation of hip, 0–2 years;
- other acute rheumatic conditions, e.g. Still's disease.

Table 10.1 • Differential diagnosis in a limping child

Condition	Systemic upset/illness	General findings	Hip movements	Walking ability	Full blood cout
Irritable hip (3–6 years)	No	Recent urti	Mild limitation	Limps	Usually normal
Perthes' disease (5–9 years)	No	Nil	Limited extension	Limps	Normal
Slipped epiphysis (9–15 years)	No	Nil	Internal rot	Limps/unable	Normal
Septic arthritis (0–10 years)	Yes	Unwell, toxic	Marked limitation	Unable	Raised

Reference to the differential diagnosis shows a number of serious conditions that may lead to permanent disability. If in doubt seek a senior opinion.

A child presenting with failure to weight bear, a limp, or pain in the hip or knee must be fully assessed and investigated

---

General assessment

History

Note the mode of onset of pain, pattern of pain, especially if the pain keeps the child awake at night. There should be a careful note of any other symptoms such as a sore throat, any other recent illnesses, the general condition of the child including appetite, presence of fever. A previous history of any other medical problems or any other joint problems should be elicited.

Examination

Note any pallor, fever, lymphadenopathy, rashes, and the general condition of the child. Check the pulse and temperature. **Look** — The position of the hip is noted. Child with significant hip pathology will often hold the affected hip slightly flexed.

Feel — The hip joint is deep and palpation can be relatively unrewarding. Examine the testes, if appropriate, since referred pain from a torsion of the testis can occasionally present with hip problems.

Move — Commence examination with movements of the **opposite** hip. Begin with gentle rotation of movements of the other leg and as confidence is gained, flex the knee and hip fully. If there is significant hip pathology then flexing the **non-affected** hip will cause apparent increase in the flexion of the affected hip (Thomas' test, (Fig. 10.2).

Movements of the affected hip are then tested. Major findings of hip pathology include a flexion deformity at the hip, trying to bring the hip into neutral causes pain and also rotations of the hip are reduced, specifically internal rotation. Restriction in movement may be surprisingly slight even with severe pathology such as slipped epiphysis, but, in general, severe pathologies tend to cause major limitation in movement and severe pain on movements.

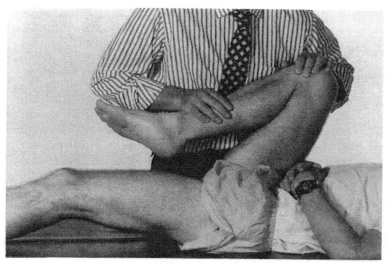

Fig. 10.2 ● Thomas' test. The opposite hip is flexed and the abnormal hip rises up, revealing the flexion deformity.

If the child is not in severe pain then the child should be observed walking.

Investigations

The plan of investigations will depend on the clinical picture and examination findings. X-ray is definitely indicated in the older age group to exclude a slipped epiphysis or if Perthes' disease is suspected. In the 2–6-year-old age group ultrasound may be the investigation of choice since this is the most sensitive method of diagnosing a hip effusion, a common finding in irritable hip. Child's temperature, full blood count, and ESR are indicated in undiagnosed causes of hip pain.

Sepsis (Softer)

Septic arthritis

An ill child, presenting with pain and inability to weight bear should be referred for a senior opinion.

Epiphyseal and childhood problems (softEr)

Perthes' disease

The patient is in the 5–9-year-old age group. An ultrasound scan may indicate an acute effusion. X-ray may be normal in the initial stages, but flattening, sclerosis, or collapse of the femoral head may be seen. Any child presenting with an unexplained limp should be referred for a further opinion.

Slipped upper femoral epiphysis

> **This condition is often misdiagnosed in A&E departments**

The patient is an adolescent and often presents with pain in the knee. There may be a history of some minor episode of trauma, this is not usually severe in nature and may not be directly associated with the onset of symptoms. There may be a surprisingly good range of movement of the hip but extremes of movement will be painful.

X-rays including a lateral view of the hip are taken. The diagnosis may be difficult. Fig. 10.3 outlines the characteristic findings on X-ray.

If there is doubt in the diagnosis in an adolescent presenting with hip or knee pain then a senior opinion should be sought (Box 10.1).

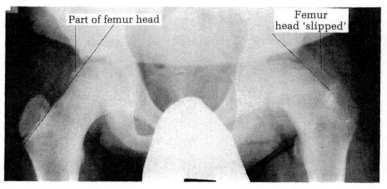

Part of femur head

Femur head 'slipped'

Fig. 10.3 • Slipped upper femoral epiphysis. Check that a line drawn along the neck of the femur passes through the femoral head epiphysis (compare with other side).

Box 10.1 • What would the senior do?

- Take a full history of the pain, the mode of onset, progress, other symptoms.
- Take a full paediatric history.
- Examine the child, generally noting temperature, etc.
- Examine the back/abdomen.
- Examine the other hip.
- Examine the affected hip.
- Watch the child walk (if possible).
- X-ray the hip including a lateral view (or 'frog lateral').
- Refer the child to orthopaedics if there is continuing or increasing symptoms.

Seronegative arthritis (tisSues) — reactive arthritis — 'irritable hip'

The child is usually 2–6 years of age with a history of a limp or non-weight bearing. There is often a history of a recent upper respiratory tract infection, but the child is otherwise well.

General examination

The child is well and temperature is normal.

Examination

The hip may be remarkably normal, but there is usually some restriction in movement. Observe the child walking.

Investigation

In a typical case ultrasound is the investigation of choice. This will show a hip effusion.

Treatment

If the child is well with no systemic upset, a normal temperature, normal ESR, and white-blood cell count, then they may be allowed home with advice to rest. They should be reviewed in an appropriate clinic in 2–3 days time.

Non-trauma — hip pain, adults (SOFTER TIsSueS)

Pain in the hip/buttock/thigh with no history of trauma is a very worrying symptom. Pain is commonly referred from the back, pelvis, or abdomen to this area. A full history should be taken. Full examination of the back, hip, and abdomen (including rectal examination) may be necessary as well as a vaginal examination. If these examinations are negative, the X-rays reveal no acute pathology, the patient is apyrexial and systemically well they may be referred to their GP for further investigations.

Sepsis (Softer)

The increasing number of patients with prosthetic hips has led to an increase in the incidence of osteomyelitis in this region in elderly patients. This complication should be suspected in a patient with a prosthesis who presents with an increase in pain. Refer such patients to the orthopaedic team for full assessment.

Osteoarthritis (sOfter)

This is an extremely common cause of hip pain. Several different patterns of hip joint disease are described, but the common symptoms and findings are of pain on walking (may be referred to thigh/knee) and stiffness with reduction in internal rotation and extension.

Patients do not commonly present with stable arthritic symptoms and a sudden increase in symptoms, disability, and signs may indicate complications (sepsis, fracture) or other pathology.

Fractures (soFter)

The problems associated with fractures of the neck of the femur are discussed above (p. 180). Minor pelvic fractures, trochanteric avulsions are often seen in the elderly. Good quality X-rays should be obtained in patients presenting with a recent onset of hip pain or an increase in hip symptoms.

Stress fractures of the pelvis or hip may be found in young, fit athletes or very active individuals.

The most common joint surgery involves the hip. While most of these operations are highly successful and cause few problems, associated complications include loosening of the prosthesis, dislocation, erosion of the acetabulum, and infection. Patients with a joint prosthesis and an increase in symptoms should be fully assessed, good-quality radiographs obtained (ensure that the X-ray shows the area below the prosthesis), and orthopaedic review organized.

Tendon, muscle, and deep bursa (sofTer)

Adductor tendinitis

Most common in horseriders and athletes. There is specific tenderness at the insertion of the adductors into the ischium. Treatment is rest in the initial stages and then a gradual return to training, preferably under the direction of a physiotherapist. The muscle may rupture and operative repair is sometimes advised.

Rupture biceps femoris

This occurs in young, fit individuals after a sudden contraction of the quadriceps. There is tenderness over the anterior inferior iliac spine, pain on resisted knee extension and passive hip extension. X-ray may show avulsion of a bony fragment. Surgical repair may be considered in top-class athletes.

Trochanteric bursitis and gluteal tendinitis

The patient often presents with severe pain over the greater trochanter. There is localized tenderness over the upper part of the trochanter. There is pain on external rotation with the hip flexed. X-ray may show calcium deposition within the tendon (a form of calcium pyrophosphate tendinitis).

Treatment for a typical calcific tendinitis is steroid injection into the deposit (as for supraspinatus tendinitis at the shoulder). For less acute or chronic problems, rest and analgesia are recommended and the patient reviewed by the GP.

Epiphyseal and childhood problems (softEr)

These problems are outlined in the section on the limping child.

Referred pain and neural compression (softeR)

Pain from the abdomen, aorta, pelvis, and back may be referred to the hip. Especially in the elderly, a detailed history and examination and appropriate investigations may be required to exclude problems requiring urgent treatment.

> **Consider referred pain in any patient with non-traumatic hip pain**

Meralgia paraesthetica

This condition is caused by compression of the lateral cutaneous nerve of the thigh, usually as it emerges through the deep fascia at the level of the anterior superior iliac spine. Most commonly there is no precipitating trauma, but occasionally there can be a history of a blow to this area.

The patient complains initially of pain and paraesthesia in the region of the distribution of the nerve on the outer, upper aspect of the thigh, which eventually subsides leaving a numb area that may be permanent.

No specific treatment is given for this condition, but they may be referred to their GP for follow-up if required.

Other conditions to be considered (TIsSuEs)

T pelvic secondaries;
I ischaemia of the buttocks/aortic occlusion;
S Reiter's disease, reactive arthritis;
E Paget's disease (the hip and thigh are the commonest sites of Paget's disease).

Further reading

1. Brenkel, I. J., Prosser, A. J., and Pearse, M. (1986). Slipped capital epiphysis: continuing problem of late diagnosis. *British Medical Journal*, **293**, 256–7.
2. Corrigan, B. and Maitland G. D. (1994). *Musculo-skeletal and sports injuries*. Butterworth–Heinemann, Oxford.
3. Cyriax, J. H. and Cyriax, P. J. (1993). *Cyriax's illustrated manual of orthopaedic medicine* (2nd edn). Butterworth–Heinemann, Oxford.
4. McRae, R. (1990). *Clinical orthopaedic examination* (3rd edn). Churchill Livingstone, Edinburgh.
5. Paice, E. (1995). Pain in the hip and knee. *British Medical Journal*, **310**, 319–22.

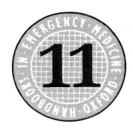

CHAPTER 11

The knee

Key points

- Anatomy
  - Major weight-bearing joint.
  - Depends on ligaments and muscle power for stability.
  - Injuries often damage ligaments leading to instability.
  - Injuries always limit muscle power leading to instability.
  - Normal ROM-flexion 135 degrees, extension 0 degrees to 10 degrees hyperextension.
- Injury
  - Refer intra-articular fractures, haemarthroses, mechanically unstable knees to orthopaedics.
  - Arrange review for traumatic effusions.
  - Rupture of quadriceps tendon/patellar tendon may be missed if straight-leg raise is not tested.
- Non-trauma
  - True giving way and locking indicate an intra-articular loose body.
  - Functional giving way indicates quadriceps weakness
  - **Beware referred pain from hip**.

Anatomy and function

The area around the knee contains a complex of joints, ligaments, and supporting muscular structures. The joints consist of the knee joint proper, between the distal end of the femur and upper tibia, the patellfemoral joint, and the superior tibiofibular joint.

The bony contours of the knee impart little structural stability to the joint. Knee stability is highly dependent on muscle power. Many minor knee symptoms are due to muscle weakness, symptoms such as 'functional giving way' must be distinguished from true 'giving way' which indicates significant structural damage to the menisci, the ligaments, or a loose body within the knee.

Definition of symptoms

Periarticular swelling — Generalized swelling around the knee joint but no demonstrable effusion.

Effusion — Swelling within the knee joint.

Bony swelling — Definite hard swelling attached to bone.

Functional giving way — Very common symptom due to weakness of the quadriceps muscle or interference with extensor mechanism. Patient describes the knee as feeling weak, often snapping into extension going up and down stairs. This is a common symptom in anterior knee pain and in any condition causing quadriceps weakness.

True giving way — This is caused by a mechanical derangement within the knee. The patient gives a clear history of walking along and they are suddenly thrown to the ground because the knee has let them down. This usually signifies a torn cruciate ligament loose body or displaced, torn meniscus.

True locking — The patient gives a history of being unable to straighten the knee into full extension. This again usually signifies mechanical derangements such as a loose body or displaced torn meniscus.

The main structures surrounding the knee are shown in Fig. 11.1.

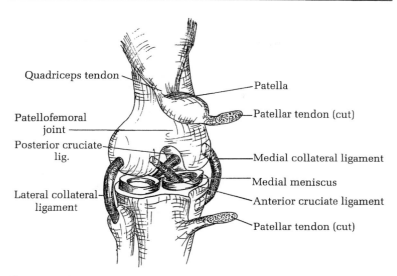

Quadriceps tendon

Patella

Patellofemoral joint

Patellar tendon (cut)

Posterior cruciate lig.

Medial collateral ligament

Medial meniscus

Lateral collateral ligament

Anterior cruciate ligament

Patellar tendon (cut)

Fig. 11.1 ● Highly schematic diagram of the knee.

Muscle power

Quadriceps and other muscles are the most important structures providing functional stability around the knee joint. The
quadriceps arises from four heads from the pelvis and femur
and is inserted through the quadriceps tendon into the patella
and from the patella through the patellar tendon into the tibial
tuberosity. The extensor mechanism is an extremely common
source of knee symptoms, including functional giving way
and anterior knee pain (chondromalacia patellae). During
simple activities such as going up stairs, forces on the joint
between the patella and femur may equate to 3.5 times that of
bodyweight (Fig. 11.2).

Other muscles around the knee include the hamstring
muscles (semi tendonosis, semi membranosis, biceps femoris),
and the smaller thigh muscles sartorius and gracilis. Popliteus
and gastrocnemius muscles also assist in maintaining the stability of the knee.

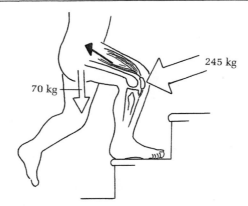

Fig. 11.2 ● Patellofemoral loading. When going up stairs 3.5 times the bodyweight goes through the patellofemoral joint.

The medial and lateral collateral ligaments

The medial ligament is a strong structure comprising superficial and deep components and runs from the medial epicondyle of the femur to the tibia, being inserted approximately 4 cm below the joint line. The lateral collateral ligament runs from the lateral epicondyle of the femur to the head of the fibula.

The collateral ligaments help to maintain the stability of the knee to lateral stresses. The commonest mechanism of injuring these structures is by a heavy blow to the body or leg while the leg is bearing weight.

The commonest injury is to the medial collateral ligaments since blows to the outer side of the leg and knee are much more common than those to the inner aspect of the knee.

Cruciate ligaments

The anterior cruciate ligament runs down from the lateral femoral condyle forwards to the region of the anterior tibial spine. The posterior cruciate ligament runs from the medial femoral condyle to the posterior tibial spine. These ligaments help to maintain anteroposterior stability of the knee joint.

They become less taut when the knee is flexed and also when the tibia is rotated laterally on the femur. Tears of the anterior cruciate ligament are the commonest cause of acute haemarthrosis in the injured knee. Twisting injuries of the knee and anteroposterior forces may cause damage to these ligaments.

The menisci

The medial and lateral menisci act as 'elastic washers' that help spread the load from the femoral condyles to the tibia, thereby lessening impact forces. They also contribute to joint stability. Because of their vulnerable position between the grinding force of the femur and the flat tibial condyles, these structures are susceptible to both acute tears and chronic degenerative damage. Any loss of substance of the menisci will increase the stresses on the femur and tibia, reducing the 'shock absorption' function of the knee and leading to greater stresses on articular cartilage. If pieces of the menisci become detached or misplaced they can act as loose bodies within the knee joint.

Examination

Assessment

General examination

Note the general body habitus of the patient, make sure that the patient is comfortable and relaxed. Check the pulse and temperature in cases of non-traumatic knee pain.

Joint above — The hip is examined and moved. Note the bulk of the quadriceps muscle.

Look — Observe any swelling around the knee or any bruising, erythema, or scarring. If there is swelling around the knee, this is probably the best time to check if the swelling is due to a knee effusion.

A *knee effusion* is demonstrated by using either the *patellar tap test* or by *cross fluctuation*. With either test, the suprapatellar pouch is emptied using one hand to move any fluid from the suprapatellar pouch down into the knee joint proper.

An effusion may then be demonstrated by tapping the patellar against the femoral condyle (Fig. 11.3). Cross fluctuation is performed by again emptying the suprapatellar pouch and then using the other hand to empty either the medial or lateral joint compartment and then stroking the opposite joint compartment while observing for fluid bulging into the empty compartment (see Fig. 11.3).

Feel — Commence palpation away from the painful area. Landmarks are more easily felt with the knee flexed to approximately 90 degrees. Palpate up the lateral aspect of the tibia until the finger falls into the joint line, just lateral to the patellar tendon. The finger can then progress around the joint line until the joint line becomes indistinct. This marks the point where the lateral collateral ligament crosses the joint line and the fibula and femoral attachments can be palpated out at this time. Posterior to the collateral ligament, the joint line is

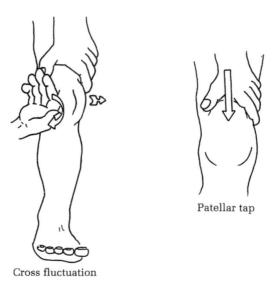

Patellar tap

Cross fluctuation

Fig. 11.3 • Knee effusion. Milk the fluid from the suprapatellar pouch into the knee joint. Then tap down on the patella or use the cross fluctuation method (e.g. for small effusion).

rather indistinct, but the tendons of the biceps femoris are felt outlining the lateral boundary of the popliteal fossa.

Palpate up the medial border of the tibia until the finger falls into the anterior part of the medial joint line, just medial to the patellar tendon. This is the point of attachment of the anterior horn of medial meniscus and the coronary ligaments. Palpate around the joint line again until the joint line becomes indistinct. This marks the point where the medial collateral ligament crosses the joint line (Figs. 11.4A,B).

Behind the medial collateral ligament lie the tendons of semitendinosis and sartorius. Palpate the extensor mechanism commencing at the tibial tuberosity, proceeding superiorly over the patellar tendon, the patellar quadriceps tendon, and the quadriceps muscle belly. Palpate the popliteal fossa and artery,

Move

Passive range of movement. Gently assess the passive range of movement. Note extension of the knee, not only the range of movement but the 'end feel' of this movement. Often limited extension will be due to pain and muscle inhibition secondary to haemarthrosis and effusion. This may be overcome by distracting the patient to allow further muscle relaxation and further extension is possible. However, if there is a mechanical block to extension, such as a loose body or displaced cartilage, the 'end feel' will be rubbery and bouncy. Note the degree of flexion possible. Note the degree of great pain experienced by the patient within the extremes of range of movement. In a haemarthrosis there is often marked pain on any movement.

Active range/resisted movement. Ask the patient to lift the leg off the couch to test straight-leg raising. If the patient is unable to do this due to pain, gently lift the leg, while supporting the heel, and then ask the patient to take the weight off the leg. If the patient is unable to straight-leg raise, then this signifies potential damage to the quadriceps tendon, the patella itself, or the patellar tendon.

The inability to straight-leg raise also occurs in very painful knee conditions such as haemarthrosis.

Stress testing — Stress testing of ligaments in the acutely injured knee is a difficult and often misleading examination.

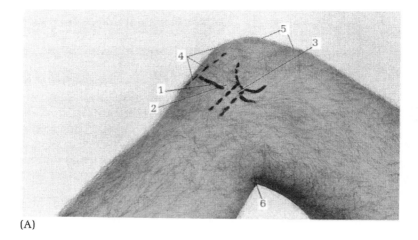

(A)

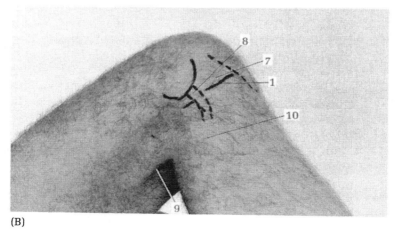

(B)

Fig. 11.4 ● (A,B) Knee palpation. Use a single finger and palpate each of the structures shown and described in the text. Upper surface of tibial condyle (1), medial joint line (2), medial collateral ligament (3), patella and patellar tendon (4), quadreceps and quadreceps tendon (5), semi membranosis/semi tendonosis tendons (6), lateral joint line (7), lateral collateral ligament (8), biceps femoris tendon (9) and head of fibula (10).

The major determinant of knee stability is muscle power and, in the acutely injured knee, reflex muscle spasm can greatly inhibit the ability of the examiner to demonstrate ligamentous instability. Care and gentleness and the use of techniques to distract the patient's attention can assist in carrying out these examinations. *Collateral ligaments.* When testing the collateral ligaments the knee must be flexed to 15–20 degrees. When the knee is fully extended, other ligaments are taut and the knee may appear stable even if there is a complete tear of a collateral ligament. The control of thigh rotation is difficult when carrying out this manoeuvre, and it requires some experience. Methods of carrying out these tests are shown in Figs 11.5A.

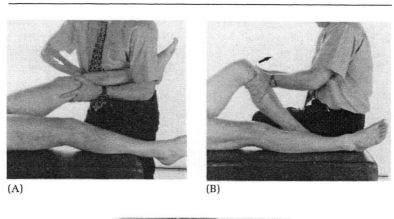

(A)   (B)

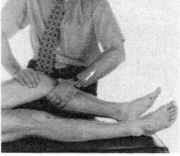

(c)

Fig. 11.5 ● Stress testing the ligaments. The patient must be relaxed. (A) Medial collateral; (B) anterior draw (C) Lachmann's.

There may be a significant degree of normal laxity especially when testing the lateral ligament. Assess the range of movement, the degree of pain felt by the patient, and the 'end feel' of movement. There should be a good solid 'end feel' of this movement. If the ligament appears lax then compare with the non-injured side. A Grade 1 tear will have a definite end point while a Grade 3 injury will be lax with an 'empty' end feel.

Cruciate ligaments. Laxity of the posterior cruciate ligament can be demonstrated by placing the pelvis level on the examination couch and flexing the knees to 90 degrees, with the heels level. By looking across the tibial tuberosities there is a posterior sag of the tibia if the posterior cruciate is ruptured.

Anterior cruciate ligament. This can be tested in a number of ways. All of these tests may be difficult to carry out in the acutely injured knee. *The anterior draw test* is performed with the knee flexed to 90 degrees and the foot stabilized by the examiner. The tibia is pulled forward on the femur and the degree of laxity noted. The same test can be carried out on the other side for comparison and also the same test can be carried out with the tibia internally and externally rotated (Fig. 11.5B).

Lachmanns test. The thigh is supported by a blanket and the knee held at 20–30 degrees of flexion. The degree of anterior movement of the tibia is checked by pulling forward on the tibia and stabilizing the thigh with the other hand (Fig. 11.5C). Other tests are described such as pivot shift test, but this can be very difficult to apply to an acutely injured knee.

Function — If the patient is badly injured then it may be impossible to observe them walking or crouching. However, for more minor injuries or for more chronic problems, it is important to observe the patient walking, crouching, and, if possible, going up and down stairs.

Nerves and vessels — As with all injuries distal neurovascular function must be checked. This can be done by palpating the pulses ensuring that foot dorsiflexion is present and that toe plantar flexion is present.

Investigations

X-rays are usually indicated in the acutely injured knee. Although the positive yield may be low, missing a significant fracture in the major weight-bearing joint can lead to catastrophic consequences. The two standard views are the horizontal beam lateral and the anterioposterior. The horizontal beam view will reveal the presence or absence of a haemarthrosis shown as a fat-fluid level just proximal to the patella (see Fig. 11.7). Other views may be indicated depending on the mechanism of injury and suspected pathology:

- A sky line view of the patella in direct blows to the patella.
- An intercondylar (tunnel view) if a loose body, or osteochondritis dissecans is suspected.
- Oblique views if a tibial plateau fracture is suspected.

Trauma — acute knee injury

Assessment & treatment

History

A clear picture of the *mechanism of injury* is essential in the diagnosis of acute knee injuries. This gives the clinician an accurate idea of the direction and strength of forces applied to the structures around the knee (see Fig. 2.2).

The *progress* and *duration* of symptoms may indicate the severity of damage. Injuries with immediate disability and immediate inability to weight bear indicate a more severe spectrum of damage to knee structures.

Past medical history is important since there are certain pathologies, such as a loose body or meniscal tear, that require referral for appropriate orthopaedic management.

Treatment

Accurate diagnosis in the acutely injured knee is difficult. Even experienced orthopaedic surgeons will reach an accurate clinical diagnosis in only 7 cases out of 10. Fig. 11.6A shows a simple algorithm for the management of such injuries.

If the disability and swelling commenced *immediately* after injury then there is likely to be a haemarthrosis. At least 70 per cent of haemarthroses will have significant mechanical injuries

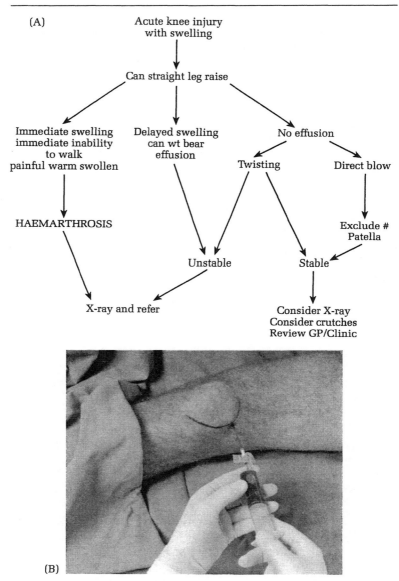

(A)

Acute knee injury
with swelling

Can straight leg raise

Immediate swelling
immediate inability
to walk
painful warm swollen

Delayed swelling
can wt bear
effusion

No effusion

Twisting

Direct blow

HAEMARTHROSIS

Exclude #
Patella

Unstable

Stable

X-ray and refer

Consider X-ray
Consider crutches
Review GP/Clinic

(B)

Fig. 11.6 ● (A) Algorithm for the management of acute knee injury. (B) Aspiration of the knee joint. Use strict aseptic technique and local anaesthetic. The lateral part of the joint is approached in the space between the proximal lateral border of the patella and the femoral condyle. Use an intravenous cannula.

to the knee, thus orthopaedic referral is indicated either immediately or to the next fracture clinic depending on local protocol.

If the swelling has been delayed then orthopaedic referral may still be indicated if there are signs of instability around the joint or if blood is found on aspiration of the joint. (Joint aspiration may be indicated in A&E depending on local protocols (Fig. 11.6B). If the knee appears to be stable, there are no signs of haemarthrosis, and X-rays are normal then the patient may be treated conservatively. This treatment would consist of assisting weight bearing using crutches, some form of simple support, elevation, and the application of ice. Exercise is encouraged with graded exercises to improve mobility, strength, and proprioception. The patient is followed-up, this could be either in the A&E clinic, a fracture clinic, or by the local GP depending on local protocol.

Trauma — collateral ligament injury

Collateral ligament tear

History

This is a common sporting injury with a valgus force being applied to the knee often with the patient weight bearing — disability may be immediate or delayed.

Examination

Look — There is swelling (bruising may appear after 1–2 days) over the medial aspect of the knee. Usually no effusion. If an effusion is present then other structural damage is possible. In a complete tear of the medial collateral ligament the joint capsule will be breached and there may be no effusion within the knee.
Feel — There is very specific tenderness over the medial collateral ligament often at the point of femoral insertion.
Move — Extension is normally limited by about 5–10 degrees. Flexion is very limited, seldom can the knee be flexed more than 90 degrees. There is pain on stressing the medial collateral ligament and there may be signs of laxity.
Function — Patients with Grade 1 (stable) injuries can usually walk, but they keep the knee as straight as they can to avoid any rotational stresses.

Investigations

X-rays — These are usually normal. In chronic medial collateral ligament problems there may be calcification near the insertion of the ligament to the femur (Pellegrini–Stieda lesion).

Treatment

Grade 1 — Simple support, early mobilization, and physiotherapy if a high level of activity is needed.
Grade 2 — May require crutches, simple support or knee brace, physiotherapy, and follow-up.
Grade 3 — If an unstable knee is suspected refer to the in-patient orthopaedic team.

Lateral collateral ligament injury

History

A varus stress to the knee, although most common in sport, this injury is also seen in motorcycle accidents and car accidents.

Examination

Look — There is swelling over the lateral collateral ligament.
Feel — There is tenderness over the ligament, very often at its midpoint or at the fibular attachment.
Move — Extension may be limited by 5–10 degrees, flexion limited to 90 degrees. There is pain on stressing the lateral collateral ligament. Try to assess stability.
Nerves and vessels — Ensure normal function of the common peroneal nerve (foot dorsiflexion is present).

Investigations

X-rays — These are usually normal. Check there is no fracture of the fibular head.

Treatment

Grades 1–3 are managed the same way as for medial collateral ligament injuries (see above).

Trauma — cruciate ligament injury

Anterior cruciate ligament tear

History

This is often a twisting, weight-bearing injury on the flexed knee, a common sporting injury, and the commonest cause of haemarthrosis.

Examination

Look — The knee is swollen and an effusion is present.
Feel — Tenderness can be hard to elicit, tenderness over the medial collateral ligament might indicate damage to both structures.
Move — Knee movements will be very limited due to effusion. Knee extension will be limited by 20 degrees or more. Flexion is rarely possible past 90 degrees. Anterior draw or Lachmann's test may show increased anteroposterior movement.

Investigations

X-rays — These may be normal, may show a lipohaemarthrosis, or may show an avulsion of the anterior tibial spine.

Treatment

If a haemarthrosis is present treat according to the local protocol, this may be by immediate referral for an orthopaedic opinion or by aspiration, support, crutches, and review in the next fracture clinic.

If there is no haemarthrosis follow the guidelines on p. 204.

Trauma — meniscal injury

Assessment and treatment

History

This is often a twisting weight-bearing injury on a flexed knee, and is a common sporting injury. More minor mechanisms of injury can give rise to meniscal tears if there is pre-existing degenerative change.

Examination

Look — There is often an effusion.

Feel — There may be specific tenderness over the joint line, but this can be hard to elicit if the tear is posteriorly placed.

Move — There will be characteristic limitation in knee movement due to acute effusion. Pay particular attention to the 'end feel' of passive extension rather than the typical 'doughy' 'end feel' of an effusion, there may be a rubbery mechanical block to full extension. This could indicate that the knee is truly locked (i.e. unable to extend) due to a displaced meniscal fragment.

Classical tests for meniscal tear (such as McMurray's test) can be very difficult to perform on the acutely injured knee.

Function — If weight bearing is possible then observe the patient walking and crouching.

Treatment

Refer to orthopaedics if the knee is truly mechanically locked. If not then an early (2–7 day) outpatient appointment is desirable.

Trauma — extensor mechanism injuries

Dislocated patella, quadriceps tendon rupture, patellar rupture, patellar tendon rupture

Dislocated patella

This injury is commonest in young women. The patella almost always dislocates laterally, often with surprisingly little trauma. The dislocation often reduces before the patient is seen, but if it is still present then gentle pressure on the lateral aspect of the bone usually effects the reduction. If this is the first dislocation experienced by the patient then the knee is immobilized using a Plaster of Paris cylinder and the patient referred to the fracture clinic. Recurrent dislocations may be treated by a simple support bandage and the patient seen in the fracture clinic.

Ruptures of the extensor mechanism

These injuries are usually caused by forceable contraction of the quadriceps muscle. The most common is rupture of the quadriceps just above the patella. This usually occurs in an elderly patient with a history of a minor stumble or fall. Patellar tendon rupture is most common in young, fit individuals exerting maximum force through the extensor mechanism (e.g. high jumpers).

Examination

Look — The knee may appear generally swollen but there may be no effusion. The patella may be 'high riding' (appear to sit more proximally than usual).

Feel — There is tenderness over the affected structure. In the elderly the tenderness is most commonly felt above the patella, in the young it is over the patellar tendon. There may be a palpable defect.

Move — Straight-leg raising must be tested on every knee injury otherwise these injuries will not be diagnosed

---

Investigations

X-ray may be normal. If damage to the patella is suspected, obtain a sky-line view. In a patellar tendon rupture, the patella will be placed much more proximally than normal.

Treatment

The patient is referred to the orthopaedic team for operative management.

Non-trauma — knee symptoms and assessment

General assessment and treatment

The common presenting symptoms to an A&E department in a patient with non-traumatic knee problems are:

* knee pain;
* knee swelling;
* giving way or locking.

> **Any patient presenting with pain in the knee but with no signs of knee pathology and no history of trauma should have their back and hips examined**

Knee symptoms are common and normally do not indicate serious pathology. However, in a small minority of patients, symptoms might indicate significant mechanical problems in the knee or even limb-or life-threatening pathology such as sepsis or tumour.

History

A careful history is the key to the diagnosis in these problems. The character, type, duration, and radiation of any pain should be noted along with the mode of onset of the pain and subsequent progress. Record any previous knee problems or knee injuries, type of employment, and sporting activities. Enquire regarding the patient's previous medical history, any medication, and any previous joint problems.

Examination

General examination — Should note the patient's colour, any rashes, the presence of other joint problems, the patient's weight, height, and record the temperature and pulse. The patient should be undressed.

Box 11.1 • Diagnoses and symptoms in non-traumatic knee pain (**H**, heat; **S**, swelling; **E**, effusion; **GW**, giving way; **L**, locking

S Bursitis (**H, S**), septic arthritis (**H, S, E**)
O Osteoarthritis (**S, E, L, GW**)
F Missed tibial plateau, patellar or ostochondral fractures (**S, E, L, GW**)
T Anterior knee pain and other patellofemoral problems (functional giving way)
E Traction apophysitis (Osgood–Schlatter, etc.)
  Osteochondritis dissicans (**E, GW, L**)
  Referred pain from slipped upper femoral epiphysis
R Referred pain from hip and back

T Osteosarcoma (**S**)
S Rheumatoid (**E**)
S Reiter's disease, other seronegative arthropathy (**S, E**)
U Gout and calcium pyrophoshate arthropathy (**H, E**)
E Rickets and Paget's (**S**)

Look for signs of quadriceps wasting and any other deformities or swelling around the knee. Examine the abdomen, back, and hip for any signs of pathology.

Feel — Check if there is any temperature difference between the knees (if the patient is wearing a bandage there may be a slight temperature difference). Elicit the exact points of tenderness.

Move — Examine all movement including active and passive range, resisted movements, and stress testing.

Function — Observe the patient standing, walking, sitting, and, if possible, crouching.

Nerves and vessels — Vascular and neurological assessment are especially important in the assessment of these problems.

Investigations

These will be entirely dependent on the clinical history. X-rays are often normal, but they may reveal missed fractures, loose bodies, or a tumour. If there is any increase in heat, if the patient is unwell, if there is a suspicion of a more generalized arthritic process then white-blood count, ESR, and a rheumatological screen may be necessary.

Treatment

Management will depend on the individual most likely cause. However, if sepsis and a serious cause of referred pain, e.g. slipped femoral epiphysis, or pain caused by neurological abnormalities can be excluded, then the patient may be properly referred back to their GP at an early stage for further assessment, investigation, and, if necessary, specialist referral.

Non-trauma — sepsis (Softer)

Bursitis, septic arthritis, osteomyelitis
Acute prepatellar and patellar bursitis are common problems in A&E medicine. Many of these will be inflammatory rather than infective, but it can be hard to differentiate between infection and inflammation on clinical grounds.

Septic arthritis and osteomyelitis are extremely uncommon, yet the importance of these diagnoses means that they should be considered in any patient presenting with an acutely painful, swollen knee.

Differentiation of bursitis joint/bone sepsis

History

Patients with prepatellar or infrapatellar bursitis usually present with a gradual onset of symptoms over 1–2 days with increased pain on walking, swelling of the knee, and limping. There may be an occupational history such as carpet-laying or increased kneeling.

Examination

The signs of prepatellar, infrapatellar bursitis are typical and normally allow a confident clinical diagnosis to be made of a bursitis.

Look — In bursitis the swelling is limited to the prepatellar or infrapatellar area. *There is no knee effusion.* There is often significant surrounding erythema and the area is hot. The patient is not generally systemically unwell, although they may have a mild pyrexia a high temperature is extremely uncommon.

Feel — There will be localized tenderness around the bursa. There will be little tenderness around the other structures of the joint and no bony tenderness.

Move — Movements will be restricted, but it is usually easy to flex the knee from 0 to 60 degrees without too much pain. Past 60 degrees, pressure on the bursa increases and flexion becomes increasingly painful.

Investigation

Further investigation is not usually merited unless there is doubt regarding a diagnosis or if there is a suspicion that there may be a penetrating injury and a retained foreign body.

Treatment

Bursitis is very painful and often initially disabling. However, it responds very quickly to treatment with rest (crutches required), elevation, an anti-inflammatory agent and an antibiotic are prescribed. The patient should be reviewed within 24–48 hours and by this time the condition is usually settling. Uncommonly, an abscess forms in the bursa and this may very occasionally require incision and drainage.

Septic arthritis/osteomyelitis

History

The patient is often unwell. There is a history of severe pain, especially at night, often with constitutional symptoms such as high temperature, fever, nausea, and vomiting. Weight bearing is very difficult or impossible. In a child it may be a refusal to weight bear on that limb.

Always ask about a history of a recent penetrating injury or medical procedure (e.g. aspiration, joint replacement, steroid injection).

Examination

Look — The patient looks unwell and has a high temperature. The knee is held in about 20 degrees of flexion. Note any evidence of joint penetration or scars.
Feel — The knee is hot and there is an effusion within the knee (septic arthritis). There is generalized tenderness. Any movement of the knee is exquisitely painful.

Investigations

A full blood profile and ESR are performed, X-ray is taken.

Treatment

The patient is referred immediately to the orthopaedic team for further care and assessment.

Note

In osteomyelitis the signs may be much more subtle. The patient again is generally unwell and there is severe pain keeping him awake. The patient may, however, be able to weight bear, there may be tenderness confined to one of the bones, this may or may not be erythema. If this diagnosis is in doubt then a full blood count and ESR are obtained and a senior opinion requested.

Osteoarthritis and degenerative arthritis

Assessment and treatment

The knee is one of the commonest joints to be affected by osteoarthritis. This is especially common in the joint between the patella and the femur. Degeneration may also affect the menisci leading to problems such as effusions, loose bodies, and locking. Unless there has been some specific knee trauma in the past, patients with degenerative disease of the knee are normally over 30 years of age.

Examination

Findings on examination are largely unremarkable. There may be some evidence of deformity, usually valgus deformity, osteophytes may cause marked swelling.

Treatment

Symptomatic treatment is given. The patient is encouraged to exercise up to the limit of pain, especially to maintain good quadriceps bulk and function. The patient is referred to the general practitioner for continuing treatment.

Osteoarthritis and effusion

Osteoarthritis is a very common cause of a knee effusion. This may be due to the arthritis itself, but complications such as loose body need to be excluded.

History

There is often a previous history of knee problems with pain and stiffness. History of locking or giving way may indicate a need for further investigations.

Examination

There is usually a small or moderate effusion, there is no increase in heat, and there is a surprisingly good range of movement. The patient can usually weight bear reasonably well. If there is a history of locking or giving way then X-rays may be required to exclude a loose body, otherwise they may be referred back to the GP for further care and assessment.

Non-trauma — fractures and osteochondritis

Missed fractures

Although many knee fractures are obvious on the initial radiographs a significant number may be overlooked, these are shown in Fig. 11.7A. The small osteochondral fracture and the tibial plateau are the most difficult to see on initial X-rays.

Alternatively, the precipitating incident of trauma may have been many years previously. A detailed history should be

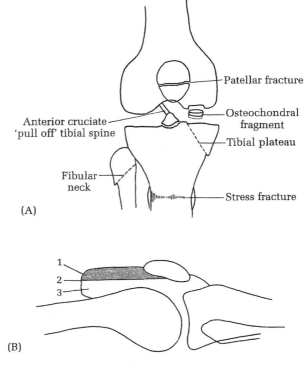

(A)

Patellar fracture

Osteochondral fragment

Anterior cruciate 'pull off' tibial spine

Tibial plateau

Fibular neck

Stress fracture

(B)

1
2
3

Fig. 11.7 ● (A) Missed fractures around the knee.
(B) Lipohaemarthrosis; Fat (1) floats on blood (3) giving a fluid level (2).

taken noting the previous trauma and, if possible, old notes
and X-rays should be reviewed. Old fractures may cause symptoms due to osteoarthritis or due to loose body formation.

Osteochondritis dissecans

This is a condition in which loose osteochondral fragments
separate from the femoral condyle.

History

The patient is in their teens or early twenties and presents
with pain, an effusion, and perhaps giving way or true
locking.

Examination

Confirms the effusion, but little else may be evident unless the
knee is locked.

Investigations

X-ray — These should include an intercondylar view if the
condition is suspected (see Figs. 11.8).

Stress and pathological fractures

These fractures may occur in the upper tibia or lower femur in
the elderly, especially in those with joint replacements.
Ensure that X-rays show the bone beyond the stem of any
prosthesis.

Non-trauma — tendon and muscle problems

Apart from the localized swelling of Osgood–Schlatter's
disease the presence of a knee effusion should raise suspi-
cions of greater significant pathology than the more benign
diagnosis of mechanical knee pain.

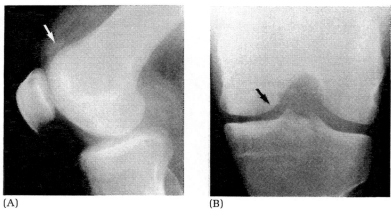

(A)   (B)

Fig. 11.8 ● Osteochondritis dissecans. The fragment has separated from the inner aspect of the femoral condyle and is acting as a loose body in the suprapatellar pouch.

Anterior knee pain (chondromalacia patellae)

This is one of the commonest knee problems. The patient is often a teenage girl or young woman who gives a characteristic history of pain over the anterior aspect of the knee which is worse on exercise, especially when climbing stairs. There is a history of functional giving way (a feeling that the knee is insecure). There is no history of previous knee trauma, general health is good, and there is no night pain.

Examination

Look — There are often no abnormalities to be seen, although there may be some mild quadriceps wasting.

Feel — There is no increase in temperature. There is often generalized tenderness around the knee and especially over the patella. There may be tenderness on the undersurface of the patella.

Move — There is usually full range of movements. There may be a catch pain through a range of flexion, but normally full extension and full flexion can be achieved. In severe cases, severe muscle inhibition causes very marked limitation of movement. Ligaments here are stable. Straight-leg raising is of good power and is normal. The patellar-grinding test is a rather non-specific test said to be positive in this condition. The patella is compressed against the femur and the patient asked to contract the quadriceps muscles. This results in pain in the affected area (compare with other side).

Function — Often the patient can walk well but there is pain going up stairs. Gait analysis may demonstrate excess pronation of the foot leading to altered mechanics at the knee. Foot orthoses may be indicated after biomechanical assessment.

Investigations

Usually no investigations are necessary in a typical case. However, if there are abnormal findings and atypical features (effusion, night pain, true giving way, or locking), then X-rays may be required (including skyline view).

Treatment

Treatment of these cases can be difficult and is normally outside the scope of A&E practice. Physiotherapy will ensure good quadriceps tone and there are various taping and strapping regimes that are said to give relief to these symptoms. Whatever methods or treatments are advised the patient should be assured that there is no serious pathology within the knee, that this is a common problem, and normally it will resolve with time. The patient may then be referred to the care of the GP for continuing care and assessment.

Non-trauma — epiphyseal and childhood problems

Traction apophysitis

In children aged between 5 and 15 years of age the knee is the commonest site of traction apophysitis. Osgood–Schlatter's disease affects the tibial tuberosity, but there are minor variants of this along the course of the extensor mechanism from the upper pole patella, the lower pole patella, and tibial tuberosity.

History

The history and findings are usually very characteristic. The child is usually very active, often playing a lot of sport and there is pain over the anterior aspect of the knee on exercise.

Examination

Look — There is often no abnormality seen, although there might be some slight swelling of the tibial tuberosity.
Feel — There is specific tenderness at the site of the affected apophysis, this could be the upper pole patella, lower pole patella, or tibial tuberosity.
Move — There is full range of movement of the knee, but there is pain on resisted extension.

Investigations

X-ray — If the findings and history are typical then X-ray is not normally required. (If the point of tenderness is not over the expected site then X-ray may be required.)

Treatment

The child and parents are given a clear explanation of the cause of these symptoms. The symptoms often settle with a period of enforced rest, especially from sport, and the patient is referred to the GP for review and follow-up.

Osteochondritis dissecans

This disorder may affect older children. There is separation of an osteochondral fragment from the femoral condyle (Fig. 11.8).

History

There may be an episode of minor trauma that precipitates the attendance. Often with pain, limping, and swelling.

Examination

An effusion is apparent.

Investigations

Standard views may miss this lesion. Intercondylar views are requested in addition to the standard projections.

Osteomyelitis and septic arthritis

In the past these knee disorders were almost exclusively childhood problems, but while this is now less common in children the increasing numbers of prosthetic knee joints has led to an increase of osteomyelitis in the elderly.

Fractures

Children have very specific types of fractures around the knee that may not be spotted on initial assessment. Small osteochondral flakes, although innocuous on X-ray which shows only a very small slither of bone, often result in sizable cartilaginous fragments being removed from the articular surface. This can cause problems with secondary degenerative changes and loose body formation.

Non-trauma — referred pain, the hip

In a patient presenting with knee pain and no swelling, the the hip, back, and abdomen should be examined.

Apart from sepsis, there are a few other causes of severe pain that may require immediate diagnosis and action. However, slipped upper femoral epiphysis and some causes of back or abdominal pain referred to the leg may require urgent treatment (aortic aneurism, cord compression).

Non-trauma — tumour

The area around the knee is the commonest site of presentation for primary osteocarcinoma, this typically occurs in the

10–20-year-old age group. The patient presents with pain and swelling. However, normally there is no effusion. The swelling is over the bone and there is normally a slight increase in temperature. A patient presenting with a bony swelling and knee pain should be given an X-ray. If no swelling is present, the patient may be referred to the GP for early review and consideration for a subsequent X-ray.

Seronegative arthritis

Assessment and treatment

This is one of the commonest joints involved in reactive arthritis.

History

Take a very full history in such patients. In addition to the standard questions regarding the presenting symptoms ask about other symptoms such as sore throat, upper respiratory tract infection, eye problems, back problems, bowel symptoms, or genitourinary symptoms.

Examination

A general examination should be carried out for stigmata of systemic disease and the general health of the patient. Specific examination of the knee seeks to elicit any signs that may suggest a septic arthritis (see above).

Investigations

Full blood count, ESR, and rheumatological screen may be necessary along with specialized investigations that may be indicated after clinical examination (e.g. MSU, back X-ray, rheumatoid factor, urate).

Treatment

Any patient presenting with such an acute arthritis should be referred to a rheumatologist or orthopaedic surgeon for further assessment and follow-up.

Non-trauma — gout

Assessment and treatment

Gout and psuedogout are common in the knee joint and the surrounding bursae. The presentation may be difficult to differentiate from septic arthritis, with a very painful, hot stiff joint.

History

This may reveal a previous history of gout or risk factors for gout. Exclude any history of joint penetration or operations on the knee.

Investigations

If there is any doubt regarding the diagnosis then the joint should be aspirated and the fluid sent for microscopy to exclude microorganisms and to confirm the presence of crystals. X-ray may show chondrocalcinosis within the menisci making a diagnosis of pyrophosphate arthropathy much more likely.

Endocrine/metabolic problems

While swellings around the knee due to rickets are now rare in current practice in the United Kingdom, this diagnosis will be missed if it is not considered. Epiphyseal swelling, bony deformity, and muscle weakness are the presenting symptoms.

Rarely other metabolic disease such as acromegaly or hypothyroidism may present with a knee effusion.

Pitfalls how to avoid them

- Arrange referral/review for significant knee injuries in patients with high functional demands.
- Tibial plateau and small osteochondral fractures are easy to miss — refer all haemarthoses.

- Quadriceps/patellar tendon injuries are easy to miss. Refer all patients who cannot straight-leg raise.
- Consider referred pain in patients with no local signs.

Diagnoses not to miss:

- *Acute septic arthritis.* Think of this diagnosis in a patient with no history of trauma and a hot knee with an effusion.
- *Referred pain from hip* (especially the elderly and the child or adolescent). Always examine the hip in these age groups and arrange appropriate X-rays if hip movements are painful.
- *Referred pain from serious abdominal pathology.* If there are no local signs examine the abdomen, especially in women where gynaecological pathology may cause obturator nerve irritation.
- *Occult fractures.* Always suspect a fracture if there is a lipohaemarthrosis visible on the X-ray. Examine the tibial plateau carefully. Obtain special further views such as tunnel views, obliques, sky-line views as indicated by the clinical assessment.

Further reading

1. Griffin, L. (1995). *Rehabilitation of the injured knee* (2nd edn). Mosby, St Louis, Missouri.
2. Johnson, ... (1993). Anatomy and biomechanics of the knee injuries. In *Operative orthopaedics* (2nd edn), (ed. M.W. Chapman), pp. 2039–54. J. B. Lippincott, Philadelphia.
3. Larson, R. L. and Burger, R. S. (1993). Medial instability of the knee. In *Operative orthopaedics* (2nd edn) (ed. M. W. Chapman), pp. 2115–30. J.B. Lippincott, Philadelphia.
4. Packer, G. L., Gainer, A. D., Cracksford, A. D., Coll, A. M., and Goring, C. C. (1992). Effect of an algorithm on the treatment of knee injuries. *Injury*, **23**, 270–2.
5. Schenck, R. C. and Heckman, J. A. D. (1993). *Injuries of the knee* Ciba–Geigy, New Jersey.
6. Steadman, R. J. and Sledge, S. L. (1993). Non operative treatment and rehabilitation of knee injuries. In *Operative orthopaedics* (2nd edn) (ed. M.W. Chapman), pp. 2055–62. J.B. Lippincott, Philadelphia.

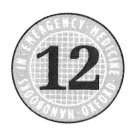

CHAPTER 12

The leg

Key points

- Trauma
  - The tibia and fibula are commonly fractured, even by a seemingly innocuous blow (e.g. a kick when playing football).
  - Compartment syndrome is commonest in the leg. Suspect this in a patient with severe pain following injury.
  - Haematomas may be tense enough to compromise skin vascularity.
  - A patient with a sudden sharp pain behind the heel has a rupture of the Achilles tendon until proven otherwise. All such patients must have Simmond's test (or similar) performed.
  - In children, fractures of the tibia are very hard to diagnose. Suspect in a toddler who is not weight bearing after a minor twisting injury.
- Non-trauma
  - Suspect deep venous thrombosis in non-traumatic calf pain.
  - Stress fractures of the tibia and fibula are not uncommon.

Anatomy

The major function of this area is weight bearing and locomotion. Injuries or pathologies in this area, if not correctly diagnosed, can severely affect the patient's long-term mobility and level of function.

The tibia and fibula form the bony skeleton. Most of the medial border of the tibia is easily felt beneath the skin (shin bone). The head of the fibula is felt easily below the joint line of the knee but is rather indistinct, covered with muscles, until approximately 9–10 cm above the lateral malleolus. The bones are joined by superior and inferior talofibular joints and a strong interosseous membrane.

The muscles of the leg are divided into 4 groups, each with its separate fascial compartment (Fig. 12.1). The extensor muscles lie lateral to the subcutaneous border of the tibia, these include the tibialis anterior and the extensor muscles of the toes. Peroneal muscles overlay the fibula. At the back of the calf there are 2 compartments: the superficial compartment, containing the soleus and gastrocnemius; and the deep compartment, with the tibialis posterior and flexors of the toes.

The 2 main nerves supplying this area are the common peroneal nerve and the tibial nerve. The common peroneal nerve is at risk of injury over the head of the fibula.

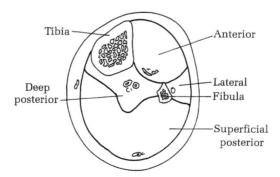

Fig. 12.1 • Cross-section of the leg to show the fascial compartments surrounding the muscle groups. Increase of pressure in these compartments will cause compartment syndrome.

Trauma — pain in anterior leg

Fractures of tibia and fibula, acute compartment syndrome, subcutaneous haematoma.

Fractures

Fractures of the tibia and fibula are common, even after mild to moderate trauma such as a kick while playing football. In toddlers, a minor twisting injury may cause a spiral fracture. Radiography is indicated to exclude such fractures. In the child the fracture may be very difficult, if not impossible, to spot on the initial X-ray. Seek an early review in such cases.

Acute compartment syndrome

Muscle groups are contained in tight myofascial compartments (see Fig. 12.1). An acute injury will cause swelling and bleeding into this compartment with a resultant rise in pressure. As the pressure rises blood flow will be reduced, producing critical ischaemia of the muscle group.

The lower leg is one of the commonest sites for this problem. Direct blows, crushing injuries, and fractures of the tibia (often undisplaced), may cause this syndrome. Compartment syndrome may also occur in patients with bleeding disorders or in those taking anticoagulant drugs.

This is a surgical emergency as any delay in relieving the pressure will result in muscle necrosis with subsequent major disability.

The diagnosis is made on clinical grounds. The main presenting feature is of severe pain. It is more common following crush injuries, but may be seen after fractures or during reperfusion of ischaemic tissue and occasionally in the absence of any acute episode of injury. The patient complains of severe unremitting pain that is keeping them awake and which is made worse by any attempt to move the foot either actively or passively.

Examination shows marked tenderness over the affected muscle groups and *pain on passive stretch of the affected muscle groups.*

> The diagnosis of acute compartment syndrome is made on clinical grounds. Any patient with severe unremitting pain following injury to lower leg should be referred

The diagnosis of compartment syndrome is entirely compatible with normal pulses in the foot and normal sensation in the foot. Treatment of this condition is outside the scope of the A&E department but all cases must be recognized and the patient referred to the inpatient team.

Subcutaneous haematoma

Direct blows to the lower limb often cause significant bruising, especially in the elderly. This may be severe and take the form of a subcutaneous haematoma. The diagnosis is made from the history of an injury along with the findings of a tender, painful swelling in the subcutaneous tissue. The swelling is fluctuant.

Most of these injuries can be treated conservatively. Occasionally, the pressure within the haematoma is so intense that it can cause necrosis of the overlying skin. If the haematoma is large and tense, and especially if there is blanching of the skin over the apex of the swelling, then the whole of the haematoma should be incised and drained. This may require a general anaesthetic and it is also wise to leave a drain within the haematoma cavity otherwise the haematoma simply re-forms.

Trauma — sudden pain in the calf

Ruptured Achilles tendon, tear of calf muscles, Baker's cyst and deep venous thrombosis

Ruptured achilles tendon

History

The patient complains of a of sudden, severe, sharp pain at the back of the heel while walking or playing sport. The patient is generally 35–60 years of age. The patient can still walk.

Examination

Look — Soon after injury there may be little swelling or bruising.

Feel — There is tenderness over the Achilles tendon. There may be a palpable gap, but this is not always present.

Move — The long flexors of the toes will still provide enough power to plantar flex the foot. This will be painful and weak. The patient will be unable to go up onto tiptoe. In all cases of sudden calf pain a Simmonds test must be performed.

Even with a complete rupture of the Achilles tendon the patient can still actively plantar flex the foot

---

Simmonds' test

Box 12.1 ● Simmonds' test

The patient lies prone with the ankles over the end of the couch. The alternative is to have the patient kneeling on a chair. The calf muscles on both sides are squeezed and the degree of plantar flexion of the foot is noted. If there is no or very little plantar flexion, the Achilles tendon must be assumed to have been ruptured and the patient is then referred for a senior opinion (Fig. 12.2 A,B).

Treatment

If a tear of the Achilles tendon is suspected, then seek senior advice, refer to inpatient team. Options include Plaster of Paris with the foot in plantar flexion, or surgical repair of the tendon. In most A&E departments this decision will rest with the orthopaedic department.

Tears of the calf muscles (medial head gastrocnemius)

History

The history is one of pain in the back of the calf while performing some activity, (common in badminton) and the patient normally has trouble weight bearing.

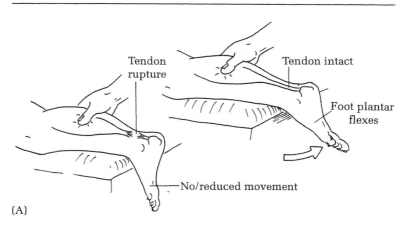

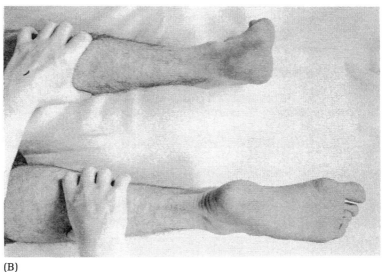

(B)

Fig. 12.2 • (A,B) Simmonds' test. In a rupture of the Achilles tendon the foot will not plantar flex when the calf is squeezed.

Examination

There is characteristic tenderness over the medial head of gastrocnemius in the mid-and upper calf. **Always ensure that the tendo-Achilles is functioning**.

Treatment

The condition normally resolves spontaneously after a 3–4-week period, but early physiotherapy can aid this process. Crutches and a heel raise may be necessary to improve patient mobility.

Ruptured baker's cyst and DVT

A Baker's cyst is a synovial cyst in association with the knee joint, usually found in patients with degenerative arthritis of the knee. This may rupture suddenly causing intense pain in the calf. The tenderness and swelling is more diffuse than in the Achilles tendon rupture or gastrocnemius rupture; it can be difficult to differentiate the condition from a deep venous thrombosis and the patient may need Doppler studies or a venogram to make the correct diagnosis.

Non-trauma — pain in leg/calf

Sepsis, fractures, tendon and muscle problems, tumour, ischaemia/DVT, endocrine

Sepsis (Softer)

Cellulitis can occur at any age, but it is more common in the elderly especially those with vascular problems or skin ulceration. It can be very difficult to treat and if there is extensive cellulitis the patient should be admitted for intravenous antibiotics.

Osteomyelitis is a rare disease, but areas around the knee and ankle are the commonest sites for this condition. Patients are often young, present with severe pain with no specific history of trauma (or a history of trivial trauma), and often they cannot weight bear. In the early stages, examination may be unremarkable or be confined to some slight erythema overlying a point of extreme bony tenderness. The patient is usually pyrexial, white-cell count and ESR are usually raised but may be normal in the early stages of the disease.

Fractures (soFter)

Stress fractures can occur in either the fibula or tibia. They are commonest at the proximal and distal ends of the bone and are characterized by the history of onset of pain with no real mechanism of injury (although there may be a history of a recent excessive use or increase in training schedules). There is tenderness over the bone and pain on stressing the bone. X-rays may be negative up to 3 weeks following the onset of symptoms. The diagnosis therefore is essentially clinical. If this diagnosis is suspected then further review is advised. The patient is advised to rest and if the pain is severe they may be given crutches to assist with weight bearing.

Stress fractures may also occur in the elderly due to poor bone quality. Diagnosis is dependent on meticulous history taking and examination, specialized tests such as bone scanning may be required to confirm a clinical diagnosis.

Tendon and muscle problems (SofTer)

Shin splints, chronic compartment syndrome, medial tibial syndrome, paratendinitis, tendon degeneration
The leg is a common site of overuse syndromes and mechanical stress problems. Although these are most common in the athletic population, they can occur in any individual who has increased their level of activity.

Diagnosis is dependent on meticulous history taking and examination, and specialized tests may be required to confirm some of the diagnoses.

'Shin splints'

This syndrome is characterized by pain over the anterior muscles of the lower leg especially on exercise. The causes include *chronic compartment syndrome* (due to an increase in compartment pressures on exercise) and the *medial tibial syndrome* (a condition with features of an enesthesiopathy at the origin of the deep posterior compartment muscles from the tibia; the condition is most often seen in those participitating in sport on artificial surfaces such as 'Astroturf').

The sufferer is usually a sportsman who gives the characteristic history of pain which on exercise is felt over the shin and reduces after a period of rest.

On examination, there may be very little to find at rest. Occasionally, there is tenderness over the inner aspect of the tibia, at the site of the muscle insertions, this is more common in the medial tibial syndrome. If there is significant swelling, pain or tenderness, especially if there is pain on passive plantar flexion and resisted dorsiflexion, then acute compartment syndrome must be considered (see above).

The patient may be given advice such as the necessity for high-quality footwear and the avoidance of a sudden increase in activity. Otherwise, investigation is normally outside the scope of A&E practice, but specialized centres may arrange bone scans or even exercise intercompartmental monitoring, and in some athletes detailed gait analysis may be required.

Extensor tendon paratendinitis

There is often a history of a sudden increase in activity with pain normally experienced over the lower anterior part of the leg. Examination is characteristic with swelling over the extensor muscles, just above the ankle joint, localized tenderness at this point often with crepitus on plantar/dorsiflexion of the ankle joint. The condition normally responds well to rest and to a non-steroidal anti-inflammatory agent. However, if there is marked pain then crutches to help weight bearing may be indicated or, in extreme cases, Plaster of Paris immobilization.

Achilles tendinitis and paratendinitis

The patient presents with a history of pain and swelling of some weeks' duration, often made worse by exercise.

Examination reveals swelling along the course of the tendon, with pain on resisted plantarflexion and passive dorsiflexion of the ankle.

Simmonds' test confirms the continuity of the tendon

The diagnosis can be confirmed by an ultrasound scan. Rest, a heel raise, and physiotherapy may help. Inexperienced staff should not give steroid injections in this area. The patient is referred to the care of the GP for further treatment.

Tumour (Tissues)

The area around the knee is the commonest site of primary osteosarcoma. The commonest age for presentation is 10–20 years. This is an uncommon tumour (the average district hospital might expect to see 1 or 2 cases per year, less than 10 per cent will present initially to an A&E department).

If a child presents with pain, bony swelling, and bony tenderness, then an X-ray should be taken to exclude this diagnosis.

Ischaemia/vascular insufficiency

Ischaemia/compartment syndrome, deep venous thrombosis
The lower leg and foot is the most common part of the body to be affected by ischaemia, vascular insufficiency, venous problems, and compartment syndrome, therefore a vascular cause should be sought in patients with pain of a non-traumatic origin. A clear history is again the key to accurate diagnosis. Severe unremitting pain suggests critical ischaemia or compartment syndrome. Pain only on walking or activity may indicate claudication, whereas a dull aching pain in the calf could indicate a deep venous thrombosis.

Rest pain and critical ischaemia

The patient often presents with a long history of vascular insufficiency, but the pain has become much worse and keeps the patient awake at night and is unrelieved by analgesics.

Examination

Look — The foot may be redder than the other side, especially in dependency. However, if the foot is elevated then the foot will blanche quickly and the veins will empty (guttering). On return to the dependent position it will become hyperaemic or cyanotic and the veins in the foot will become empty.

Feel — The affected limb may feel colder than the other. Tenderness may be generalized.
Move — All movements may be painful. Pain on passive movements of certain muscle groups may indicate critical ischaemia of that muscle group. Patients with signs and symptoms suggestive of critical limb ischaemia should be referred for immediate vascular surgical opinion.
Nerves and vessels — It is essential that the femoral, popliteal, and pedal pulses are palpated carefully. If no pulsation is felt then blood flow may be checked using a Doppler probe.

Intermittent claudication

The history is usually very characteristic. Pain is felt in the calf on exercise and relieved after a period of rest. The distance the patient can walk is usually constant. A full medical history is taken, noting any risk factors for vascular disease. Examination methods are listed above under rest pain and *critical ischaemia*.

Patients who have stable intermittent claudication but no increase in symptoms should be referred back to their GP for further management. They may require further investigation and treatment on an elective basis.

Deep venous thrombosis

This is one of the commonest diagnostic problems presenting in the lower limb. Table 12.1 lists some important clinical points that may differentiate between patients at high risk of having a DVT against a low risk of DVT. With reference to Table 12.1, patients with a high clinical probability of DVT had an 85 per cent prevalence of DVT proven by venography, whereas those with low clinical probability had a 5 per cent prevalence of deep venous thrombosis.

If this model is combined with ultrasound in patients who have a low probability of DVT clinically and have normal ultrasound results this indicate that the likelihood of a proximal deep venous thrombosis is less than 1 per cent. Patients with negative scans should have a another review and scan in 3–4 days to check that a small calf thrombosis (which may be missed on scanning) has not propagated.

Table 12.1 • Pointers to the clinical risk of DVT. (From Wells P. S., Hirsh J., Anderson, *et al.* (1995). Accuracy of clinical assessment of deep-vein thrombosis. *Lancet*, **345** 1326–9)

Major pointers to DVT
- Active cancer
- Paralysis
- Within 4 weeks of major surgery
- Thigh and calf swelling on measurement
- Strong family or previous history of DVT

- Plaster immobilization
- Bedridden for more than 3 days
- Localized tenderness along the deep veins
- Calf swelling: > 3 cm greater than other side

Minor pointers
- Recent history of trauma in symptomatic leg
- Dilated veins only in symptomatic leg
- Erythema

- Pitting oedema only in symptomatic leg
- Hospital inpatient within last 6 months

Clinical risk
High — If 3 or more major factors, or 2 major and 2 minor
Low — 1 major and 2 or less minor **and** alternative diagnosis
— 1 major and 1 or less minor, but **no** alternative diagnosis
— 3 or less minor **and** alternative diagnosis

For patients not in the low-risk category then a further opinion is needed.

Extra-articular rheumatism/endocrine

Paget's disease, rickets

Paget's disease

The tibia is one of the commonest sites of the bony changes characteristic of Paget's disease. Bone pain is the commonest symptom which is often continuous and not relieved by posture or rest. Pain at night is common. There may be local tenderness and bony deformity may occur (tibia). Diagnosis is confirmed by X-ray. The patient may be referred to the GP for further care and assessment.

Rickets

Vitamin D deficiency is very uncommon in the United Kingdom. The patient is usually a young child often from an ethnic minority. They may present with walking disorders or deformity of the leg. Diagnosis is made by taking a history, examining the patient, and ordering appropriate X-rays and biochemical tests (alkaline phosphatase, calcium and phosphate).

If rickets is suspected then the patient should be referred for a paediatric assessment on an outpatient basis.

Further reading

1. Allen, M. J. (1990). Shin pain. In *Sports injuries recognition and management* (ed. M.A. Hutson), pp. 149–152. Oxford University Press, Oxford.
2. Lorentzon, R. (1988). Causes of injuries. Intrinsic factors. In *The Olympic book of sports medicine* (ed. A. Dirix, H. G. Knuttgen, and K. Tittel), pp. 376–90. Blackwell Scientific Publications, Oxford.
3. Mubarak, S. J. (1982). The medial tibial stress syndrome. *American Journal of Sports Medicine*, **10**, 201–5.
4. Mubarak, S. J. (1993). Compartment syndromes. In *Operative Orthopaedics* (2nd edn) (ed. M.W. Chapman), pp. 379–96. J. B. Lippincott, Philadelphia.
5. Renstrom, P. (1988). Diagnosis and management of overuse injuries. In *The Olympic book of sports* medicine (ed. A. Dirix, H. G. Knuttgen, and K. Tittel), pp. 446–68. Blackwell Scientific Publications, Oxford.
6. Shepherd, R. J. and Astrand, P. O. (1992). *Endurance in Sport*. Blackwell Scienctific Publications, Oxford.
7. Wells, P. H., Hirsh J., Anderson, *et al.* (1995). Accuracy of clicical assessment of deep-vein thrombosis. *Lancet*, **345**, 1326–9.

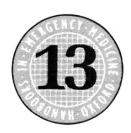

The ankle joint

Key points

- Anatomy
  - The ankle is a major weight-bearing joint which depends on muscle power and reflexes for stability.
  - Movements at the ankle joint are dorsiflexion (20 degrees) and plantar flexion (50 degrees)
  - Inversion and eversion occur at the subtalar joint.
- Trauma — ankle sprains
  - Ankle sprains are common but often undertreated.
  - 50 per cent of patients will still have some symptoms at 1 year following an ankle sprain.
  - *Expected* level of function required for a patient's occupation or leisure is important when deciding treatment.
  - Rehabilitation advice is required, even after a simple sprain.
- Other trauma
  - Falls from heights often cause severe injury.
  - Calcaneal fractures may be overlooked if specific X-rays are not taken.
  - Exclude more proximal and lumbar spine injury.

Introduction

Ankle injuries account for 5 per cent of the workload of an average A&E department. Most of these injuries will be partial tears of the anterior talofibular ligament (ankle sprain). While many sprains are self-limiting, the injury can give continuing symptoms in up to 50 per cent of patients 1 year after the injury.

The familiarity of this injury may lead to short cuts in patient management, but full patient assessment is essential and the treatment tailored to the patient's need will improve the outcome for most patients.

Anatomy

The ankle is a complex series of joints including the ankle joint proper between the dome of talus, the tibia and the fibula, the inferior tibiofibular joint, and subtalar joint between the talus and the calcaneum.

The major factor in stability of the ankle joint is strong muscle power. Loss of muscle function is the commonest cause of instability following ankle injuries. The loss of the normal proprioceptive reflexes and muscle wasting commonly lead to a feeling of instability and continued 'going over' on the ankle.

The ligaments of the ankle are shown in Fig. 13.1. The most commonly damaged ligaments are those on the lateral aspect where the capsule of the ankle joint is thickened in 3 places. The commonest injury is a partial tear of the anterior talofibular ligament. If the injuring force is of a greater magnitude or of a greater duration then the tear may continue around the capsule thus tearing the calcaneal fibular ligament and if severe enough tearing the posterior talofibular ligament.

Tears of the medial or deltoid ligament are rarer, but there is often some damage to the medial ligament or its bony attachment in simple ankle sprains. Damage to the deltoid ligament tends to give a more prolonged disability and a period of supervised rehabilitation will probably be needed.

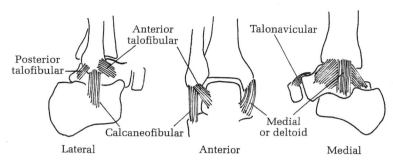

Fig. 13.1 • Ligaments of the ankle. The most common injury is to the lateral ligament especially to the anterior talofibular ligament.

Ankle movements and biomechanics

The ankle joint essentially is a hinged joint with the axis of the hinge running slightly backwards and downwards from the medial malleolus. This means that the movements of plantar-and dorsiflexion are accompanied by lateral movements of the foot. Inversion and eversion movements take place at the subtalar joint and the talonavicular joint.

Examination

Joint above — Expose both legs up to the knee joint. Palpate around the knee especially over the fibular head.

Look — Compare the limbs for any areas of bruising, swelling. Assess calf muscle bulk and tone, especially in more chronic problems.

Feel — Commence examination around the knee, paying particular attention to the fibular head as this may be fractured in severe ankle ligament injuries. Develop a routine to cover all of the anatomical structures outlined in Fig. 13.2. Palpate down the tibia, around the medial malleolus, then the medial ligament. It is quite common to detect tenderness just at the posterior aspect of the medial malleolus. Palpate the tendo-achilles, make sure this is intact. Examine the area between the Achilles tendon and the malleoli; if there is bilateral

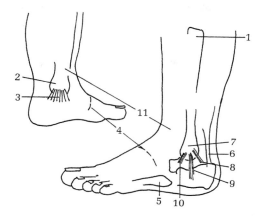

Fig. 13.2 • Palpate each of these structures carefully: 1, fibular head; 2, medial malleolus; 3, medial ligament; 4, mt–tj; 5, base of 5th metatarsal; 6, tendo-achilles; 7, lateral malleolus; 8, posterior talofibular ligament; 9, fibulocalcaneal ligament; 10, anterior talofibular ligament; 11, anterior capsule and inferior tibiofibular joint.

swelling in this area, this indicates an effusion within the ankle joint.

The foot is then palpated, especially the metatarsotarsal joints and specific attention is focused on the base of the 5th metatarsal, a common site of avulsion fractures. In most patients, examination will be negative, but failure to follow this routine will result in important injuries being overlooked. The lateral malleolus and lateral ligament area are palpated with extra care to elicit the exact point of tenderness.

Move — Active and passive movements will reveal a characteristic limitation in plantar flexion and almost absent dorsiflexion. *Resisted movements* are usually of normal power, although pain on resisted eversion is common due to tears in the invertor muscles in the calf or to avulsion injury from the base of 5th metatarsal.

Stress testing is difficult. The classical inversion stress testing is extremely painful and therefore unreliable. The anterior draw test may be helpful in confirming a complete tear of the anterior talofibular ligaments (Figs 13.3A,B), but this test is also unreliable if there is inadequate analgesia.

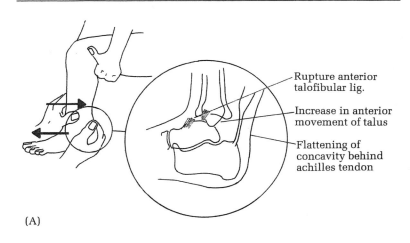

Rupture anterior talofibular lig.

Increase in anterior movement of talus

Flattening of concavity behind achilles tendon

(A)

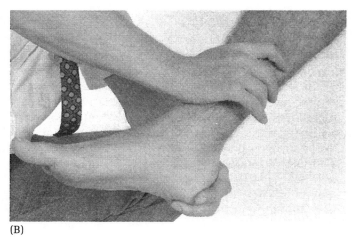

(B)

Fig. 13.3 • Anterior draw test. The muscles are relaxed (note patient supporting thigh). One hand pushes backwards on the tibia. The other hand pushes forwards on the heel. **Look** for flattening of the concavity behind the Achilles tendon. **Feel** the degree of movement and the 'end feel'. Compare to other side.

Function — If possible, observe the patient walking. In more chronic ankle problems check proprioception and muscle balance by asking the patient to stand on one leg — if they can do this, try with the eyes closed (hold the patient's hand while doing this test).

Nerves and vessels — Sensation and pulses in the foot are examined along with capillary refill in the toes.

Trauma — 'went over on ankle'

General

This history is compatible with a whole range of injuries from minor self-limiting ligament tears to major limb-threatening fracture dislocations. Careful clinical technique, followed by appropriate investigations are the key to accurate diagnosis.

History

Mechanism of injury. The exact mechanism of injury is ascertained. The commonest is that of the patient walking or running and going over on the ankle with the foot going into inversion. Other mechanisms where the forces are greater, of different direction, of greater duration should increase suspicion of a more severe injury. In a patient falling down stairs the forces are of much greater magnitude and it is difficult for the protective muscle reflexes to overcome the deforming force. Ask the patient to demonstrate the position of the ankle when it was injured (using the other ankle).

The immediate effects of injury are noted, especially if the patient could weight bear, since immediate loss of ability to weight bear should increase suspicion of a more severe injury.

Past history of injury is especially important. The current injury may be one episode in a repeated series of episodes of 'giving way'. This requires a full assessment (see below).

The expected level of activity in the patient's work or leisure pastimes is taken into account in some management discussions. Someone who depends on 100 per cent ankle stability, such as a fireman, steeplejack, or professional athlete, might need a higher level of treatment than someone who can function normally even though there is some occasional ankle instability.

Examination

If there is obvious deformity of the ankle then immediate action is essential. Fracture dislocations of the ankle commonly cause problems with the skin, and thus the limb must be placed in normal anatomical alignment. If possible, the patient should be given analgesia, preferably intravenously, supplemented by Entonox, the knee is then bent, the heel grasped and gentle axial traction applied. Figure 13.4 shows the bones placed in normal alignment. Pulses should be checked before and after this procedure.

Where there is no apparent deformity, follow the procedure above (see Examination pp. 242–5). Take care to examine all the structures at risk, and to accurately localize the tenderness to specific structures, for example it is important to differentiate between tenderness over the anterior part of the malleoli and the posterior aspect of the bone (see 'Ottawa rules' (Fig. 13.5)).

The most common findings will be localized tenderness and swelling over the anterior talofibular ligament with limitation in all movements.

Other injuries often missed are to the fibular head and the tarsometatarsal joints, therefore these areas should be examined carefully.

Investigations

Should all sprained ankles be X-rayed? Of all ankle injuries 10–15 per cent are significant fractures. Many studies have developed criteria that select patients with ankle sprains who have a very low incidence of serious fractures. The most recently evaluated rules were developed in Ottawa (Ottawa rules, Fig. 13.5). There should be local guidance on the application of such rules. If a decision is made not to X-ray the ankle, then a full clinical assessment must be made and **recorded**. The patient is advised to return if they have trouble weight bearing in 3–5 days.

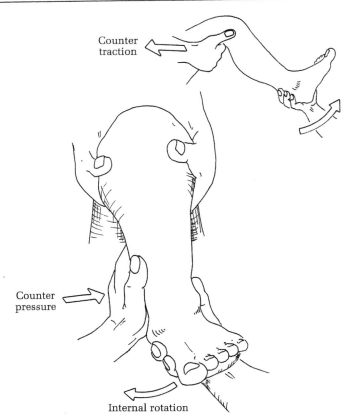

Counter traction

Counter pressure

Internal rotation

Fig. 13.4 • Reduction of dislocated ankle (external rotation type). The patient is given intravenous analgesia supplemented by Entonox. The ankle is supported while the knee is flexed. Axial traction against countertraction is applied. The deformity is then corrected by internal rotation of the foot with counter pressure over the medial malleolus.

X-ray is indicated if:

• patient is unable to weight bear immediately;
• patient is unable to walk 4 steps in A&E;
• bony tenderness as indicated in Fig. 13.5.

X-ray **ankle** for malleolar tenderness, **foot** for 5th metatarsal/ tarsal tenderness.

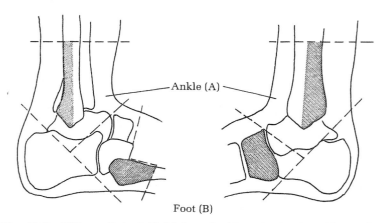

Fig. 13.5 • 'Ottawa Rules'. Guidelines for X-ray in simple ankle sprain. Bony tenderness over the points indicated requires an X-ray. X-ray is also required if the patient is unable to weight bear immediately after the accident or to walk 4 steps in the A&E department. X-ray **ankle** for malleolar tenderness and **foot** for metatarsal/tarsal tenderness. If the patient is not X-rayed then they are given instructions to return after 5 days if they have trouble weight bearing. (Adapted from Stiell *et al.*)

No clinical algorithm is 100 per cent accurate. If there are no local guidelines then the advice to the inexperienced must be to 'X-ray if in doubt'.

The normal ankle views are anteroposterior and lateral. If these X-rays are not clear then other views may be necessary, including obliques or specific views for individual bones such as the calcaneum. If there is tenderness higher up the leg, then full views of the fibula and tibia may be required. It is not necessary to routinely request ankle and foot views, however, if there is tenderness over the foot then X-rays are necessary (see Ottawa rules, Fig. 13.5).

In the simple sprained ankle, further investigations are seldom indicated. If there is any suspicion that there may be more severe injuries due to the mechanism of injury or due to clinical findings then a more senior clinical opinion is advised. Stress X-rays may be indicated, but these are unreliable in the acute injury without good analgesia. For more complex problems, then further imaging using CT or MRI may be indicated, but this is normally outside the scope of A&E practice.

Fig. 13.6 shows some of the fractures that are commonly missed on X-ray. Pay particular attention to the areas of the epiphyses in children. Fibular fractures may only be apparent on the lateral view and difficult to see due to the superimposed tibia. Small osteochondral fractures from the corners of the dome of the talus are often missed as are fracture dislocations of the metatarsotarsal joint. These are severe injuries with appreciable morbidity. Fractures of the anterior process of the calcaneum and the base of the 5th metatarsal as well as small avulsion fractures from the neck of the talus are often missed but are of less clinical importance.

Treatment

The wide spectrum of soft-tissue injury is demonstrated by ankle sprains. There can never be a 'standard treatment' for a sprained ankle. The major factors influencing treatment are the severity of injury, the functional demands of the patient, and available resources. The treatment and definition of the different degrees of sprain are described below.

Simple sprains (grade 1)

Definition

- Simple inversion injury contracted while walking/running.
- Patient can weight bear.
- The patient has no major functional demands.
- Tenderness and swelling are limited to the anterior talofibular ligament.
- X-ray (if done) is normal.

Treatment

The treatment aims are the reduction of swelling and pain and early mobilization with emphasis on achieving a normal walking pattern. This will maintain muscle strength and normal proprioceptive input.

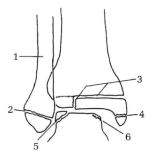

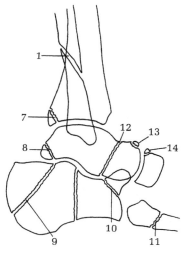

Fig. 13.6 • Commonly missed ankle fractures. 1, Oblique fracture fibula. This may be invisible on the A/P film and on the lateral the fibula is hidden behind the tibia. 2, lateral malleolus; 3, Tilleux fracture, a fracture through the distal tibial growth plate in children; 4, medial malleolus; 5, osteochondral fracture dome of the talus; 6, crush to the dome of the talus; 7, posterior malleolus; 8, posterior process of talus (do not confuse with os trigonum); 9, calcaneal fractures; 10, anterior process of calcaneum; 11, fracture base of 5th metatarsal; 12, fracture of the neck of talus (prone to develop avascular necrosis); 13, avulsion fracture from neck of talus at site of capsular insertion; 14, navicular fractures.

R, *Rest* — The patient must rest with the foot elevated above the heart to reduce swelling. After a few days they should commence gradual mobilization. They should be advised to walk normally and not on tiptoes.

I, *Ice* — Patient is advised to apply ice (in a wet towel).

C, *Compression* — This is difficult to achieve in the ankle. It can be done by properly applied strapping (see below), but most patients will probably be treated by a simple elasticated stocking bandage. This probably gives little support or compression, but patients and doctors seem to favour this type of treatment.

E, *Elevation* — Patients should be instructed to lie on the sofa with the ankle elevated on pillows.

R, *Rehabilitation* — Patients must be encouraged to walk as normally as they can, and it should be explained that this is essential to retain muscle power around the ankle joint, (see Ankle advice sheet). Physiotherapy may help in this process, but resources would soon by swamped if every sprained ankle were referred for treatment. Patients requiring a higher level of activity either in work or leisure pastimes may be referred for physiotherapy.

Moderate sprains (grade 2)

Definition

- The patient cannot weight bear.
- Swelling present over both ligaments.
- Marked swelling present.
- X-ray is normal.

Treatment

The treatment is as described above, but if the patient is unable to weight bear then they will require crutches or stick. If a walking aid is given then the patient should be formally reviewed either in the A&E department, by the GP, or by the orthopaedic department. After 1 week most patients will be walking fairly well and their symptoms will be settling. If they are still unable to weight bear then a more senior opinion is advised. Immediate physiotherapy may be beneficial to some patients with severe or moderate sprains. These patients will benefit from more formal eversion strapping such as that outlined in Fig. 13.7

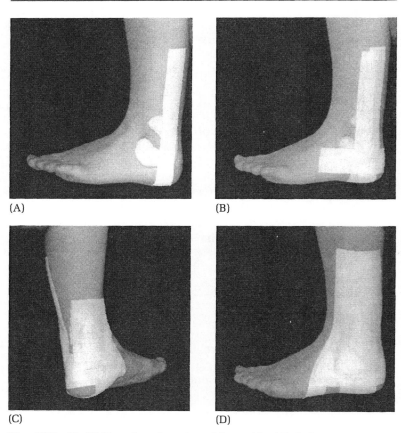

(A)   (B)

(C)   (D)

Fig. 13.7 • (A–D) Eversion strapping of the ankle. (A) Orthopaedic felt is used to apply compression to the hollows around the malleoli. A 'stirrup' zinc oxide tape is applied from the medial side up on to the lateral side of the leg with the ankle being pulled into eversion. (B) Further tape is applied at right angles to this, going around the back of the heel. The strapping is then built up by applying overlapping strips of tape. (C) As the horizontal layers lead up the leg, a gap is left at the back and a wide gap is left at the front. It is important that the zinc oxide tape is not put circumferentially around the ankle. (D) Completed strapping.

Severe sprains (grade 3)

Definition

- Severe mechanism of injury.
- Patient is unable to weight bear.
- Marked swelling and bruising present over both ligaments.
- Signs of ankle effusion present.
- Signs of instability present on anterior draw test.

Patients with severe sprains do not have self-limiting injuries, therefore they require more care and supervision in their treatment and rehabilitation. The pain is often severe and the patient may require formal support in a Plaster of Paris back slab. They will require crutches and advice regarding elevation and rest. They should be reviewed within 1 week either in the accident department consultant clinic or in the orthopaedic clinic. At that time, a further assessment is made and further investigations might be indicated (different X-rays such as obliques, foot views, stress views, or even CT scanning). Treatment options will include continued mobilization, further immobilization in Plaster of Paris, intensive physiotherapy with proper supportive strapping, or, if there is evidence of a complete tear in a patient with high demands on the ankle, surgical repair is occasionally undertaken.

Minor avulsion fractures

Small 'pull off' fractures from the lateral malleolus, cuboid, lateral aspect of the calcaneum, or the neck of the talus are common findings on X-ray. These small fragments of bone represent the insertions of the capsule of the ankle and of the ligaments. The injury is essentially a ligament injury and the treatment is determined by the factors listed above.

Complications

Functional instability

This is a common sequel in minor ankle sprains. The major complaint is that of 'going over' on the ankle, especially on rough ground. Most people have little disability, but these symptoms may interfere with leisure pastimes. The loss of proprioception and protective muscle reflexes make the ankle less able to respond to minor deforming forces. To avoid this complication patients with minor or moderate ankle sprains must be encouraged to weight bear at the earliest opportunity and to regain full muscle strength.

Mechanical instability

A minority of patients will have true mechanical instability due to a complete tear of the lateral ligament. This may be confirmed by stress X-ray with analgesia. These patients may benefit from an operative procedure to reconstruct the lateral ligament and should be referred to the orthopaedic clinic.

Missed fracture

Common sites of missed fracture are noted above, perhaps the most serious are those in children and small osteochondral fractures of the dome of the talus. These act as loose bodies in the ankle joint and may give the classical history of intermittent true giving way of the ankle joint along with ankle effusions.

Other sites of common missed injuries are the metatarsotarsal joints at the base of the 5th metatarsal and the neck or shafts of the fibula.

Peroneal tendon dislocation

If the peroneal retinaculum is torn then the peroneal tendons may slip forward over the lateral malleolus. This gives a very characteristic clinical picture, the patient complains of a snapping over the outside of the ankle on activity. These symptoms can usually be reproduced when examining the patient. This condition often responds to a period of immobilization in Plaster of Paris and referral.

Trauma — other mechanisms of injury

Hyperplantar flexion injury

The mechanism of trauma here is that the toe is caught and the ankle is forcibly plantar-flexed; it is a common footballing injury.

The major damage is to the anterior capsule and there may be small avulsion fractures from the anterior margin of the talus. These injuries can often take many weeks to settle, and a senior opinion is advised for patients who place high demands on their ankle (Box 13.1). Those patients not making good early progress may have further X-rays taken and, possibly, undergo other imaging procedures such as CT or MRI — often after consultation with the orthopaedic team.

External rotation injuries

These occur when the anterior part of the foot is caught and therefore the foot acts as a lever acting around the ankle joint. Hence, these stresses are much greater with a higher likelihood of fractures or major ligamentous disruption.

Fall from height

Falls on to the heels from a height of over 6 feet (1.83 m) should always be taken very seriously. The forces involved are of much greater magnitude. There are a number of injuries caused by this mechanism that can be hard to spot on a routine ankle X-ray.

- Examination should include the whole of both limbs and the back (lumbar injuries are common).

Box 13.1 ● What the senior would do

- Take a careful history noting all the patient's symptoms.
- Carefully examine the patient, including as routine the back, the hips and the knees.
- Request X-rays of those areas with any significant signs or symptoms.
- Check the technical quality of the films ensuring that all the relevant views are available (e.g. calcaneal, foot including true lateral).
- Consider other imaging techniques such as CT).
- Support the ankle in a wool or crepe bandage or a plaster backslab.
- Review the patient within 1–2 days.

- Note sites of specific swelling and tenderness.
- Special views may be required if the tenderness is over the calcaneum (axial calcaneal views).
- X-ray the spine if there are any symptoms or signs in the back.
- Fractures of the talus can be very hard to diagnose if adequate radiographs are not taken.
- The Tilleaux fracture is a Salter 3 injury to the distal tibial growth plate and epiphysis. This can be very hard to spot and tomograms or even CT scanning may be required to make this diagnosis.
- Patients who have fallen from a significant height and cannot weight bear should be reviewed by a senior/specialist.

Non-trauma — general

S — osteomyelitis
O — commonly post-traumatic
F — small but very important fractures are often overlooked resulting in chronic symptoms
T — Achilles tendinitis, peroneal tendon problems, extensor tendon paratendinitis, flexor hallucis longus tendinitis
E — post-traumatic, sepsis
R — referred pain from prolapsed lumbar disc

T — hypertrophic pulmonary osteodystrophy
I — DVT, arterial insufficiency
S — Reiter's syndrome
U — gout.

Introduction

In patients presenting with ankle pain and no history of trauma the same serious conditions must be excluded as in any other non-traumatic limb pain.

- sepsis
- ischaemia or vascular insufficiency
- referred pain/neural compression.

Non-trauma — pain and swelling in ankle joint

Sepsis, post-traumatic arthritis, missed fracture, seronegative arthritis, gout

An effusion within the ankle joint is diagnosed by finding swelling around the ankle, but especially in the hollows between the malleoli and the Achilles tendon. If both the medial and lateral sulci are swollen then this usually indicates an acute ankle effusion. There will be characteristic limitation of movement in a capsular pattern. Patients with signs of an effusion will require a detailed examination and investigation and a senior opinion is advised.

A full history is taken of the onset and type of pain. Any associated symptoms are noted along with a full previous history. Specific enquiry is made as in any swollen joint (see page 25).

Temperature and pulse should be recorded and a brief general examination should note the overall state of the patient. Local heat and erythema are noted, as are specific points of tenderness. The pedal pulses should be examined and a full neurological examination of the limb carried out.

Further investigation will depend on the clinical assessment. X-rays are usually indicated. A full blood count and ESR may be required.

Immediate referral is advised if the joint is hot and swollen (unless there is a clear history suggesting gout), or if there are signs of acute critical ischaemia.

Other patients should be given analgesia, support, and crutches. Review within 1–2 days should be arranged.

Non-trauma — pain in ankle, swelling not in joint

Sepsis, cellulitis/osteomyelitis, tendon problems, DVT/ischaemia/cardiac failure

Bilateral ankle swelling is common and this presentation should prompt a detailed assessment of cardiovascular function. Unilateral swelling is less common.

Cellulitis is common around the lower leg and ankle. It can often be severe and slow to resolve. Patients with large areas of cellulitis, those with *pre-existing vascular insufficiency* or with any signs of systemic involvement should be admitted to hospital for intravenous antibiotics and elevation.

One specific presentation is that of cellulitis over the medial malleolus. The patient is often young and fit with a painful hot area of erythema spreading over the malleolus. This is very hard to distinguish from osteomyelitis. If there are any systemic signs or a high pyrexia or marked night pain the patient should be admitted. If the patient is to be treated as an outpatient then they should be reviewed in the A&E department within 48 hours to ensure that the condition is settling.

Osteomyelitis is rare, but the distal tibia is one of the commonest sites. The diagnosis is difficult. **Beware** of children with severe pain in the ankle with no history of trauma (or a history of minimal trauma). Severe pain, **localized** bony tenderness, and an increase in heat over the area should prompt admission for observation and further investigations.

Tendon problems of the Achilles tendon and the foot extensors are discussed in Chapter 12.

Non-trauma — pain in ankle, no swelling

Referred pain, ischaemia

Occasionally a patient will present with severe pain around the ankle but with no local signs. *Pain referred* from the lumbar/sacral nerve roots, the hip, or the knee should be considered. Assessment of the other joints of the limb as well as a neurological examination of the limb should therefore be undertaken.

Critical arterial insufficiency will occasionally present as severe pain in the ankle. Careful assessment of the peripheral pulses is essential. Refer all such patients to the surgical/ vascular team.

Pitfalls and how to avoid them

Trauma

- *Mind set.* Ankle sprains are so common that it is very easy to get into a 'mind set' that all ankle problems with a negative X-ray are 'Simple sprains'. Adopt this attitude and you will be right 90 per cent of the time, but with an average department seeing 2500 ankle injuries per year the other 10 per cent represents 250 patients with potentially crippling pathology!
- *Missed fractures.* The mechanism of injury and the degree of disability are the main indicators of potentially serious injury. Meticulous clinical examination essential, especially of the fibula and metatarsotarsal joints. X-rays of appropriate areas needed. Check the quality, special views (obliques, calcaneal) may be needed. Fig. 13.6 shows the main area where fractures are missed. Patients unable to weight bear should be reviewed.
- *Missed rupture of the Achilles tendon.* Always check the integrity of the tendon using the Simmonds' test.
- *Missing unstable ligament injury.* Beware of medial ligament injury and inferior talofibular joint injury.

Non-trauma

- Do not miss ruptures of the Achilles tendon.
- Think of osteomyelitis in non-traumatic ankle pain.
- Think of ischaemia in non-traumatic ankle pain.
- Think of referred pain/lumbar disc.
- *Sepsis.* Consider this in a patient with severe pain and no history of trauma.

Further reading

1. Becker, H. P., Komisckke, A., Burkhard, D., Bensel, R., and Claes, L. (1993). Stress diagnostic of the sprained ankle, evaluation of the anterior draw test with and with anaesthesia. *Foot and* Ankle, 459–63.

2. Brooks, S., Potter, B. T, and Rainey, J. (1981). Treatment for partial tears of the lateral ligament of the ankle: a prospective trial. *British Medical Journal*, **282**, 606–7.

3. Chande, V. T. (1995). Decision rules for current roentgenography of children with acute ankle injuries. *Archives of Pediatrics and Adolescent Medicine*, **149**, 255–8.

4. Editorial (1989). Residual disability after ankle joint injury. *Lancet*, **1**, 1056.

5. Kelly, A. M., Richards, D., Kell, L., *et al.* (1994). Failed validation of a clinical decision rule for the use of radiography in acute ankle injury. *New Zealand Medical Journal*, **107**, 294–5.

6. Nuber, G. W. (1988). Biomechanics of the foot and ankle during gait. *Clinics in Sports Medicine*, **7**, 1–13.

7. Packer, G. J., Goring, C. C., Gayner, A. D. and Craxford, A. D. (1991). Audit of ankle injuries in an accident and emergency department. *British Medical Journal*, **302**, 885–7.

8. Raatikainen, T., Putkonen, M., and Puranen, J. (1992). Arthrography, clinical examination and stress radiograph in the diagnosis of acute injury to the lateral ligaments of the ankle. *American Journal of Sports Medicine*, **20**.

9. Stiell, I. G., Greenburgh, G. A., McKnight, R. D., *et al.* (1993). Decision rules for the use of radiography in ankle injuries. *Journal of the American Medical Association*, **269**, 1127–31.

10. Yamamoto, A., Ishibashi, T., Muneta, T., and Furuya, K. (1993). Non surgical treatment of lateral ligament injury of the ankle joint. *Foot and Ankle*, 500–4.

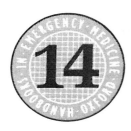

The foot

Key points

- The foot supports all the bodyweight and is essential for proper walking and running motion. It acts as a spring shock absorber through the arches of the foot. All the structures of the medial arch including all the joints of the big toe are essential for running and walking.
- Injuries to the metatarsal–tarsal joint are often severe but may be difficult to diagnose.
- Crush injury to the foot can give severe and prolonged symptoms, but X-ray appears normal. Compartment syndrome may affect the small muscles of the foot — suspect in cases of severe unremitting pain.
- Injury to the heel, such as a fall from a height, requires specific views of the calcaneum. Suspect more proximal injuries or even lumbar spine fractures in falls on to the feet from a height.
- Severe non-traumatic pain may be due to critical ischaemia.
- Stress fractures, acute gout, and hallux rigidus are common causes of non-traumatic foot pain.

Movements

- Subtalar/midtarsal joint — inversion, 40 degrees; eversion, 20 degrees
- MTPJ hallux — extension, 65 degrees; flexion, 40 degrees.
- IPJ hallux — extension, 0 degrees; flexion, 60 degrees

Anatomy

The main functions of the foot are to support the bodyweight, to provide for power transmission in walking and running, and to absorb the shocks of walking, running, jumping, etc. The basic shape of the foot is an arched spring — the heel and the area of the metatarsal heads make contact with the ground and the two arches of the foot (medial and lateral) span the gap between these two pillars (Fig. 14.1). The bony and ligamentous elements of the arches are reinforced by the *dynamic* action of the tendons. As in all joints the structure and stability of the foot depend on good muscle function and reflexes.

The most important areas in standing and walking are those associated with the medial arch especially the heel, the medial arch itself, and the big toe. Damage to these structures can give rise to a permanent disability while walking or

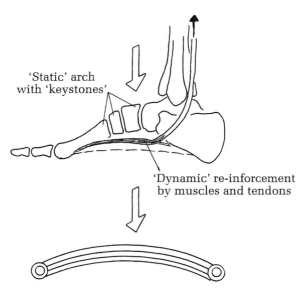

'Static' arch
with 'keystones'

'Dynamic' re-inforcement
by muscles and tendons

Fig. 14.1 • The foot resembles an arched spring with static bony/ligament structure, reinforced by dynamic muscular support.

running, and injuries to these areas need careful assessment and treatment.

Trauma — 'went over on foot'

This is a variation of the 'went over on ankle' presentation and requires a similar assessment, outlined on page X.

One fracture that deserves special mention is the fracture dislocation of the metatarsotarsal joint (MTTJ) (Lisfranc type). This is not uncommon after a simple fall downstairs. The foot is very swollen and there is specific tenderness over the MTTJs. There is pain on stressing this joint. Specifically request a true lateral of the foot if this injury is suspected. X-ray interpretation includes confirming the alignment of the second metatarsal base to the cuneiform and that no dorsal displacement has occurred (check true lateral) (Figure 14.2). Other fractures missed include those of the calcaneum, navicular, and cuneiform.

Treatment follows the usual routine of rest, ice, compression, elevation, and rehabilitation. Sprains to the metatarsotarsal joint can give fairly prolonged disability, pain, and swelling, especially in the elderly. Patients should be warned of the severity of these symptoms and, if necessary, physiotherapy organized.

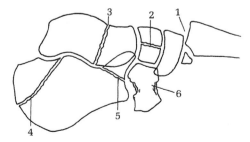

Fig. 14.2 • Missed foot fractures. 1, Fracture dislocation at the base of the metatarsotarsal joint; 2, body of navicular; 3, neck of talus (prone to develop avascular necrosis); 4, calcaneal fractures; 5, anterior process of calcaneum; 6, crush of cuboid.

Trauma — 'I dropped a heavy weight on my foot'

This is a common presentation and an accurate history and examination are the keys to diagnosis. An estimate must be made of the weight of the object and the exact mechanism of injury.

Examination records the exact areas of swelling and bruising and tenderness. Special attention is made to tendon function and neurovascular function in the toes. Passive toe movements must be tested, severe pain on extremes of passive stretch may be the sole indicator of compartment syndrome within the foot muscles. In crushing type injuries of the foot, X-rays must be taken.

Treatment depends on the severity of the injury and clinical findings.

In most cases where there is mild swelling, the patient can weight bear and general advice is given regarding elevation, the application of ice, and gradual mobilization.

Moderate and severe injuries must not be underestimated. These often give significant morbidity and it may take 3–6 weeks before the patient can return to normal activities. Advice is given regarding rest, ice, and elevation, especially on proper elevation with the patient lying and the foot elevated and supported (see p.). A patient may require crutches and a period of non-weight bearing.

If a heavy weight has been dropped on the foot resulting in a lot of swelling, pain, and tenderness, generalized over the foot and if there is pain on passive motion of the toes, then consider referral for inpatient care. *Severe pain with pain on passive stretch of the small foot muscles may indicate compartment syndrome —* **admission is essential**.

Trauma — stubbed toe

These injuries may appear trivial but they can give rise to significant morbidity lasting 4–8 weeks if the hallux is involved, then there may be more long-term problems.

Injuries of the hallux should be X-rayed. If fractures are found the area is protected from weight bearing by a meta-tarsal pad (crutches if needed) and the patient should be referred for follow-up in the fracture clinic or A&E clinic.

Injuries of the lateral toes do not necessarily require an X-ray unless there is a deformity that may require reduction. Treatment of undisplaced fractures is symptomatic.

One of the common sequelae of a stubbed big toe is a traumatic effusion or haemarthrosis into the 1st metatarsal–phalangeal joint. This is a very painful condition. There is localized tenderness and swelling over the 1st metatarsal–phalangeal joint with pain on active and passive movements of this joint. A metatarsal pad may help to give some sympto-matic relief.

Trauma — fall from height

Falls from a height should always be taken seriously. This signifies a severe mechanism of injury. Always search for associated injuries, especially in the lumbar spine/tibial plateau, and perform a meticulous examination noting specific points of tenderness.

X-ray should be taken of the foot and tarsal bones, as indi-cated by clinical examination. Specific views of the calca-neum may have to be requested. Fractures of the talus, calcaneum, navicular, and around the metatarsal–phalangeal joint can be very hard to spot on an X-ray.

> **Consider lumbar spine crush fracture in falls from height (over 6 feet (1.8 m))**

If the X-rays are normal and the patient can weight bear general advice is given. If the patient cannot weight bear then they should be given support, crutches, advice and brought back for review.

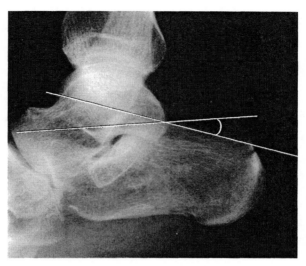

Fig. 14.3 • Calcaneal views. Bohler's angle, draw one line from the anterior process of the calcaneum through the prominence at the posterior end of the talocalcaneal joint. Draw a second line from the tuberosity through the superior prominence. The angle between these two lines is reduced when the body of the calcaneum is fractured.

Non-trauma — ingrowing toe-nail

Ingrowing toe-nail is a common presentation to A&E departments. The condition can be very painful and disabling and therefore does, at times, constitute an emergency. Treatment for this condition will depend on local protocols and some departments may not offer treatment for this condition. However, if there is marked overgrowth of granulation tissue, cellulitis, and a lot of pain then partial removal of the nail under local anaesthetic may be required. Non-urgent cases should be given advice to regularly bathe the feet in saltwater, to try and encourage the nail to 'grow out'. The best definitive treatment for this condition is to cauterize the nailbed using a strong phenol solution, but this does require meticulous attention to detail (Figs 14.4A,B)

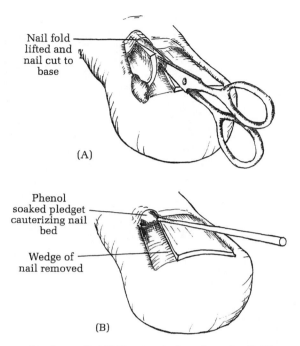

Nail fold lifted and nail cut to base

(A)

Phenol soaked pledget cauterizing nail bed

Wedge of nail removed

(B)

Fig. 14.4 • Ingrowing toe-nail. (A) Removal of wedge of nail. The nailfold is lifted up and the nailplate cut to the base. (B) Application of phenol for 3 minutes.

1. Obtain good anaesthesia by a digital block.
2. Set up all the equipment required.
3. Clean the area.
4. *Apply a tourniquet to the toe (best to use a finger cut off a surgical glove). *Note the time the tourniquet was applied.*
5. Separate the affected third of the nail from the nailbed and from the cuticle using sharp, pointed scissors.
6. Cut down the nail-plate, ensure you cut right to the most proximal part of the nail under the nail-fold.
7. Remove the wedge of nail with stout forceps using a twisting motion.
8. Ensure the area is dry with no bleeding.

9. *Apply Vaseline to all the skin around the toe to protect it from the phenol.
10. *Apply the phenol to the germinal matrix of the nail. Small pledgelets of cotton wool wrapped around an orange stick are the easiest way to do this. **Do not allow phenol to come into contact with the skin, it will cause burns.**
11. *Apply for 3 minutes.
12. *Dry the area.
13. *Wash with spirit solution to remove all traces of phenol.
14. *Remove the tourniquet — note the time.
15. Apply a non-adherent dressing and crepe bandage.
16. *Dispose of phenol safely.
17. Arrange review by GP in 3–4 days.

*Omit these steps if simply removing a nail wedge.

Non-trauma — pain and swelling, MTPJ of big toe

Osteoarthritis of 1st metatarsophalangeal joint (MTPJ) (hallux rigidus), gout/septic arthritis
Hallux rigidus is due to osteoarthritis of the 1st metatarsophalangeal joint. The history is often less acute than in gout with the patient presenting with pain and swelling of the joint and difficulty walking, but not with the same severe pain, redness, and swelling as there is in gout.

Examination shows generalized joint swelling with pain on movement, especially on dorsiflexion. If the patient is systemically well, apyrexial, and there are no other factors in the history then a non-steroidal anti-inflammatory may be prescribed, if there are no contraindications, and a metatarsal pad supplied.

Urate and crystal

A history of sudden onset of severe pain in the 1st metatarsophalangeal joint is very suggestive of *acute gout*. The main differential diagnosis to be excluded is that of *septic arthritis.* The patient may give a history of previous attacks of gout or of predisposing factors such as heavy alcohol intake, diuretic treatment.

If there is a history of a penetrating injury to the foot, then septic arthritis should be suspected. On examination, an acute gout will reveal a hot, red, tender joint with pain on all movements of the 1st metatarsophalangeal joint. The temperature is normal and the white-blood count is usually normal but may be raised. Septic arthritis will have exactly the same findings on examination, but the patient is often pyrexial and the white-cell count and ESR are elevated.

An attempt may be made to aspirate this joint but this may be very difficult. If the patient is systemically well and the history and findings indicate gout, then the patient may be given a maximal dose of a non-steroidal anti-inflammatory (for example, 50 mgs diclofenac 3 times a day for 2 days). The patient should be reviewed either by the GP or the A&E clinic in 24–48 hours. The patient is instructed that if the pain gets worse they should return to the A&Emergency department.

If there is a suspicion that the problems could be due to septic arthritis, then a senior opinion should be obtained.

Non-trauma — foot pain

Sepsis, stress fractures, epiphyseal and childhood disorders metatarsalgia, neuroma, infection, ischaemia

Sepsis

Plantar abscess, septic arthritis, septic tenosynovitis

If there is a recent history of penetrating injury to the foot then there may well be marked swelling on the dorsum of the foot, rather than the plantar aspect (similar to palmar spacing infections of the hand).

Deep infections, including tendon sheath and septic arthritis, occur following penetrating injuries to the foot.

Examination will show swelling on the dorsum of the foot. Palpation will reveal tenderness over the infected structures. If there is pain on passive movements of the joints then this should led to a suspicion of septic arthritis. Pain on extreme dorsiflexion of the toe or pain on resisted plantar flexion might indicate a flexor tendon-sheath infection.

Joint irritation is shown by great pain on any movement of the joint.

Stress fractures

The diagnosis of this injury is clinical, as X-rays taken at the time of the onset of symptoms and for up to 3 weeks afterwards may be normal. The common site is over the midshafts of the 2nd and 3rd metatarsals. If a patient presents with a recent increase in activity, localized tenderness, and swelling over the 2nd or 3rd metatarsals then stress fracture is the most likely diagnosis. Other common sites of stress fracture include the calcaneum (more common in women).

In a typical case the patient is advised that stress fracture is the likely diagnosis, they should stop their normal sporting activities or work activities if these are especially heavy. The patient is reviewed in 1–2 weeks' time to check the diagnosis. X-rays at this time may prove positive.

Epiphyseal and childhood disorders

Osteochondritis of the calcaneum (Sever's disease), navicular (Kohler's disease), and head of 2nd metatarsal (Freiberg's disease) are not uncommon.

These conditions may be asymptomatic, but chance findings on a foot X-ray taken after an episode of trauma. No specific treatment is required. The patient may be reviewed in an orthopaedic clinic or by the GP.

Referred pain and neural entrapment

Morton's metatarsalgia is due to neuroma formation in the digital nerves causing pain in the forefoot and usually radiating to the 3rd and 4th toes. Sensation may be reduced over these toes.

The posterior tibial nerve may be compressed in the *tarsal tunnel*. This gives pain and paraesthesia in the toes and sole of the foot.

Ischaemic and vascular disorders

These syndromes must be excluded in any patient presenting with non-traumatic pain. The pain is often severe, keeping the patient awake at night. Examinations are carried out as outlined in Chapter 13.

A patient presenting with rest pain and night pain should be referred *urgently* to the vascular surgical team.

Compartment syndrome can affect the small muscles of the foot. The sign is of severe pain usually following a crushing type injury with pain on passive movements of the toes. These patients should be admitted to hospital for elevation, observation, and if necessary, surgery.

Sudek's atrophy (reflex sympathetic dystrophy) is characterized by pain, stiffness, swelling, and skin changes (the skin is often shiny, red, and warm). This usually follows a period of immobility due to trauma. X-rays often show quite marked osteoporosis. The condition is difficult to treat and the patient is referred to the orthopaedic department for a further opinion.

Seronegative arthropathy

Pain under the heel

Plantar fascitis is characterized by a patient presenting with no history of trauma but with difficulty walking and pain on the plantar aspect of the foot just in front of the heel. There are very few physical signs apart from tenderness at this point. There is no swelling or erythema, all joint movements are normal. Ask about other joint problems or urinary symptoms as there is an association between plantar fascitis and Reiter's syndrome. Calcaneal spurs shown on X-ray are incidental findings and do not confirm the diagnosis.

The patient is advised to rest, a heel raise is given, and the patient referred to the GP for treatment and further investigation.

Other conditions

If patients present with undiagnosed pain in the foot with no history of trauma, and if all clinical investigations and X-rays are normal, then the patient may be referred back to the GP at an early date, as long as acute ischaemia, infection, and neural compression have been excluded.

As with any other part of the body, patients presenting with non-traumatic pain in the foot can harbour a wide variety of conditions. If the pain is severe, unremitting and especially worse at night, consider ischaemia and carefully check the pulses. Occasionally, referred pain from the back may only be felt in the foot, as might referred pain from the hip. Examine these structures.

Further reading

1. Helal, B. and Wilson, D. (1988). *The foot*. Churchill Livingstone, Edinburgh.
2. Linenger, J.M. and Shawhat, A. F. (1992). Epidemiology of podiatric injuries in USA Marine recruits undergoing basic training. *Journal of American Podiatric Medical Assocation*, **82**, 269–71.
3. Paice, E. (1995). Reflex sympathetic dystrophy. *British Medical Journal*, **310**, 1645–7.
4. Pester, S. and Smith, P. C. (1992). Stress fractures in the lower extremities of soldiers in basic training. *Orthopaedic Review*, **21**, 297–303.
5. West, S. G. and Woodburn, J. (1995). Pain in the foot. *British Medical Journal*, **310**, 860–4.

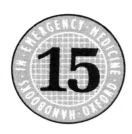

Cervical spine

Key points

- Accurate mechanism of injury is essential.
- Patients with neurological symptoms should be followed-up.
- Patients with neurological signs should be referred urgently.
- Cervical intervertebral disc protrusion may be hard to diagnose.
- Be aware of central cord syndrome developing in an older patient after a blow to the face/head.
- Many neck sprains after road traffic accidents will take 6–18 months to settle.
- Acute torticollis is a common cause of non-traumatic neck pain; often due to minor disc protrusion symptoms these often settle spontaneously in 5–10 days.
- Exclude radiation of pain from chest and heart in non-traumatic neck pain.

Introduction

Problems of the neck and cervical spine account for approximately 2 per cent of accident and emergency attendances. There is a high incidence of presentation with non-traumatic problems, a low incidence of fractures, and almost half the patients will have injured their neck in a road traffic accident. Many soft-tissue injuries of the neck give rise to significant problems that may take many months to settle. A small minority of patients will have severe damage to the soft tissues that may lead to spinal cord injury, even in the absence of any evidence of fracture or dislocation.

Anatomy

The main function of the neck is to act as a conduit for vital structures passing from the head to the trunk and to protect these structures.

The atlas and axis (C1 and C2) vertebrae are specialized to allow transmission of forces from the skull to the cervical spine and yet allow very free range of rotation and flexion extension.

The other vertebrae follow the configuration of vertebrae elsewhere in the spine, with a body, pedicles, laminae, and spinous processes.

The C1/C2 joint is highly specialized and complex. The odontoid peg (process of C2) is held against the anterior arch of C1 by its transverse ligament. These ligaments are strong and seldom injured apart from in severe trauma or if the ligament is weakened by disease such as rheumatoid arthritis. Fractures of the odontoid peg are relatively common.

The lower vertebrae have strong anterior and posterior longitudinal ligaments: the ligamentum flavum and interspinous ligament. These ligaments can be torn by moderate or severe trauma resulting in dislocation.

Apart from the atlanto-occipital joint and the C1/C2 joint, all cervical vertebrae achieve stability by the following mechanisms:

- Strong ligaments (anterior longitudinal, posterior longitudinal, interspinous, flava);

- Intravertebral discs;
- The uncovertebral joint between the *vertebral bodies* at the posterolateral margins of the vertebral body (see Fig. 15.1);
- The facet joints — these synovial joints are found at the junction of the pedicles and laminae surrounded by a joint capsule;
- Muscle power.

The vertebral column is surrounded by large muscles that may be regarded either as intrinsic muscles (taking the origins and insertions solely from the skull or cervical spine) or

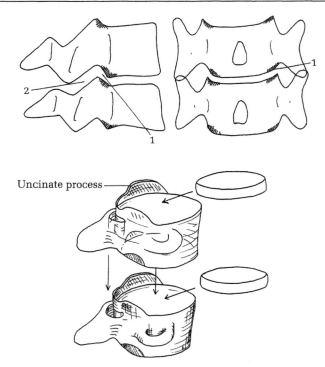

Fig. 15.1 ● The disc sits in the concavity of the vertebral body. There is a joint between the uncinate process and the lateral aspect of the vertebral body (the uncovertebral joint) (1). The facet joint is situated posteriorly (2).

extrinsic muscles (such as sternocleidomastoid, the scalene muscles, trapezius that attach the head and spine to the shoulder girdle).

The protective effect of these muscles is clearly seen in any painful neck problem where intense muscle spasm can largely prevent any neck movement. 'Muscle spasm' is a **secondary** reaction to some other painful condition; 'muscle spasm' in itself is seldom the cause of the pain.

Examination

Look — Note the position of the head, typical in acute torticollis. If the patient is holding their head 'to stop it falling off' believe them! Patients with severe bony or ligamentous injury will adopt this posture.

Feel — Carefully palpate the spinous processes looking for tenderness or gaps.

Move — This may need to be delayed until X-rays have been obtained to rule out major bony injury. In the alert patient always commence with active range. It is unlikely that a fully alert patient will allow movement that will cause more movement in an unstable injury.

The major movements are flexion, extension, lateral flexion, and rotation. There are small accessory movements of anterioposterior and lateral glide that are difficult to measure clinically. Motion is measured as shown in Figs 15.2A–G.

Lateral rotation is measured by looking down from above. Lateral flexion is the angle that the nose makes with the mid line.

The normal ranges of movement vary with age, sex, and the muscular build of the patient. In rotation 50 per cent takes place at C1/C2 with very little flexion/ extension or lateral flexion at this level. C5/C6/C7 are the most mobile areas for flexion and extension. C7/T1 is relatively immobile:

- range of flexion/extension, 120 degrees;
- lateral flexion, 70 degrees;
- rotation, 140 degrees.

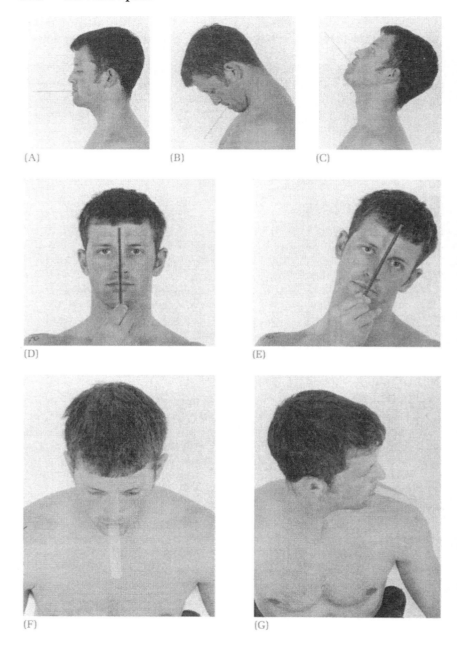

(A)

(B)

(C)

(D)

(E)

(F)

(G)

Fig. 15.2 ● Cervical spine movements. (A) neutral; (B) flexion; (C) extension; (D) neutral; (E) lateral flexion; (F) neutral; (G) rotation.

←——————————————————————————————————

These ranges will be greater in a younger person and less in the elderly.

Passive movements should not be used by the inexperienced as forceful pressure might cause serious problems.

Nerves and vessels — Neural structures and their relationships to the bony skeleton are outlined in Fig. 15.3. It is essential to test upper limb muscle power, tone, reflexes, and sensation. Also test sensation over the angle of the jaw and lower ear (C3/4) and over the occiput (C1/2).

X-ray

Cervical spine X-rays will be required in most cases of trauma. The exception to this is a patient with a typical 'whiplash' injury following a minor, road traffic accident who has full range of movement (see below).

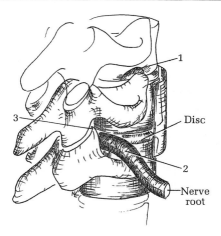

Fig. 15.3 ● The nerve root may be irritated or compressed by damage or degenerative changes around the uncovertebral joint (1), the disc (2), the facet joints (3).

In non-trauma presentations the indications are less clear-cut. The Royal College of Radiologists does not advise radiography at the time of acute presentation for symptoms typical of cervical spondylosis. X-rays are not indicated in typical acute torticollis. However, if symptoms are severe, prolonged, or if there are neurological signs or symptoms then X-rays should be taken.

Interpretation of the X-ray should follow a routine:

Quality
— Can you visualize the upper border of T1?
— Is the penetration correct, especially for visualizing the spinous processes?
— Is the odontoid peg seen clearly?

Alignment — Check all the 'lines' as shown in Fig. 15.4.

Bones — Trace around each bone in turn.

Cartilages — Check the disc spaces.

Soft tissues
— Check the width of the retropharyngeal soft tissues (Fig. 15.4).
— Check the interspinous gaps.

X-ray interpretation can be difficult, especially in the elderly with pre-existing degenerative changes and in the young. If in doubt ask for senior advice *while the patient is in the department*.

Other views

The C7/T1 junction can be very hard to image. *A swimmer's view* taken with one arm above the head and one pulled down might help check alignment at this level.

Oblique views may also assist in visualizing this area.

Flexion and extension views might be indicated if ligamentous damage is suspected. The patient must be fully alert, cooperative, and understand the procedure. *The patient must carry out these movements themselves.* A doctor should supervise the procedure, but only to tell the patient to stop if they have too much pain or any change in neurological symptoms.

Referred pain

There are two main types of pain that may be referred away from the neck into the head, lower down the trunk, or into

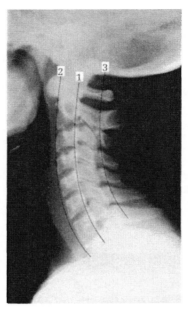

Fig. 15.4 ● X-ray of the cervical spine, the lateral (A) check the alignment of: 1, the line formed by the posterior aspect of the vertebral bodies; 2, the line formed by the anterior aspect of the vertebral bodies; 3, laminar line. Check gap between the anterior arch C1 and the odontoid. (B) Check all the bones. (C) Check the intervertebral spaces. (S) Check the width of the soft tissues and interspinous gaps.

the arm: (1) classical radiculopathy due to pressure on a nerve root; and (2) pain referred from dura, facet joints, and ligaments.

Such referred pain from non-neural structures does not conform to classical dermatomal patterns. The pain may radiate anywhere from the forehead down over the shoulders to the intrascapular area. This is important in being able to distinguish these two types of pain. The non-dermatomal pattern of referred pain from facet joints may lead to confusion and some degree of scepticism in the inexperienced. Patients complaining of such 'non-neural' referred pain usually are not overemphasizing their symptoms.

Trauma — neck pain following a minor, road traffic accident

Most patients suffering neck pain following road traffic accidents will have been involved in a *low-velocity minor impact* (less than 10 miles (16 km) per hour at impact). The patient has usually been wearing a seat belt and there has been no contact with the head and the windscreen or any other part of the vehicle.

> **Following road traffic accidents patients with neck pain caused by mechanisms of injury, other than those stated in the text must be very fully assessed including X-rays**

Neck sprain (whiplash)

This is probably the commonest reason for patients presenting to an A&E department with neck pain. While many authorities decry the use of 'whiplash', this term is very frequently used by both the public and the medical profession to describe a very definite clinical syndrome seen mainly after road traffic accidents. Readers are advised to refer to Foreman and Croft or the report of the Quebec Task Force for detailed accounts of this injury.

History

Typically, the patient will walk into the department. They will have been involved in a low-impact collision usually when their car has been struck in the rear by another vehicle. The patient is has usually been wearing a seat belt. There may be little pain in the neck at the time of the impact, but the pain gets worse over the next few hours or days and stiffness increases. The patient should be asked if there is any pain in the arms, any paraesthesia, arm weakness, a past history of neck pain, or other significant problems such as ankylosing spondylitis or rheumatoid arthritis; record all details.

Examination (in patients walking into department)

Look — There is seldom any deformity or swelling. There may be associated injury or there may be seat-belt bruising over the clavicle and anterior chest.

Feel — Tenderness is often poorly localized, involving the area over the spinous processes or more commonly in the paraspinal muscles and trapezius. Tenderness may extend up over the scalp and down to the interscapular area.

Move — If the patient is fully alert it is permissible to assess the *active* range of movements at this stage. If the patient has a fracture or dislocation it is highly unlikely that they will voluntarily move the neck to cause more damage. Passive movement, stress testing, or resisted movement are not recommended before X-rays have been obtained!

Record accurately the range of active movements, using the methods shown in Fig. 15.2. This is important as the patient's progress can be followed. There will often be limitation in all movements, but it is especially important to record directions in which rotation and lateral flexion are limited. Often there is limitation of lateral flexion to one side and rotations to the other side are more severely limited.

Function — The neck as a unit should be examined, especially noting the degree of stiffness and posture during the course of the interview.

Nerves and vessels — A full neurological examination of the arms must be carried out, noting muscle power, tone and reflexes, and checking for areas of sensory loss. It is also good practice to check the function of the lower limbs, the ability to stand on alternate legs with the eyes closed is a good screening test.

Investigations

X-ray — If the patient is fully alert, the mechanism of injury suggests a minor impact, there is no localized tenderness, and full range of movement, then X-rays may be omitted (see recommendations of the Quebec task force on whiplash-associated disorders). Patients not meeting these criteria should be X-rayed. These are often normal. However, there are some prognostic factors on X-ray (narrow spinal canal, pre-existing degenerative changes) which may indicate a more prolonged rehabilitation period, and many physiotherapists request X-rays before treating these patients to ensure there are no congenital abnormalities or other abnormalities of the spine.

Treatment

These injuries cause significant morbidity. Of patients with more minor injuries 50 per cent may have residual symptoms and up to 90 per cent of those with more severe symptoms and neurological signs may have residual symptoms (see Norris and Watts 1983).

A number of studies have shown that encouraging active-movement physiotherapy and mobilization is superior to other forms of treatment in this condition (see McKinney, Mealy). Giving a soft collar to rest the neck may help to alleviate the pain but there is very good evidence that this slows longer term recovery and prolongs the symptoms.

Patients should be given advice regarding the nature of their condition. They should be advised that trying to move the neck gently within the limits of pain is the best form of treatment, simple analgesia should be given. Patients at risk from prolonged symptoms (very stiff neck, radiation of pain to arms, pre-existing neck problems) should be referred to their GP for follow-up or referred for active physiotherapy depending on local protocols. Patients should be given advice to seek further medical help if they experience neurological symptoms in their arms or legs.

Trauma — neck injury after a fall/more severe road traffic accident

Typically, the patient is brought into the department with their neck immobilized with a hard collar and a spinal board. If this immobilization is removed then someone must be delegated to provide in-line manual stabilization of the spine at all times. Otherwise the spinal immobilization is left in place until adequate X-rays have been performed. Following an accurate history and thorough examination, including meticulous neurological examination of the arms and legs, good-quality radiographs are obtained. The interpretation of these radiographs is on p. 283.

Patients with significant mechanisms of injury and symptoms but normal radiographs are a definite diagnostic problem. There is a significant incidence of spinal-cord injury without bony abnormalities. Ligament instability, cervical intervertebral-disc protrusion can lead to progressive neural compression. All patients with neurological symptoms and signs have to be taken seriously, and referral to an orthopaedic surgeon, neurologist, or neurosurgeon may be required depending on local protocols. Definitive investigations may include CT or MRI scanning.

Neck injury in the elderly

Falls down steps or stairs are common in this age group. Fractures of the odontoid may occur (and be overlooked!). This group are at risk of developing progressive neurological signs due to *central cord syndrome*. The clinical picture is of an upper limb, lower motor neurone weakness and a lower limb, upper motor neurone lesion.

Non-trauma — Neck pain

Acute torticollis

This is probably due to a small acute intervertebral-disc prolapse. Sleeping with no support for the head places the spine in a curve which then causes pressure on the discs.

History and presentation

The classical presentation is in a patient aged 15–25 years who awakes with a stiff, painful neck. There is no history of trauma and the patient is otherwise completely well. There is usually no history of previous problems.

Other causes of such a presentation include meningitis (patient is unwell), tonsillitis, and pneumonia.

Examination

Look — The patient holds their head in a characteristic position (Fig. 15.5).
Feel — There is some tenderness over the paraspinal muscles and protective muscle spasm is easily felt.
Move — Movements are restricted and resisted.
Nerves and vessels — Full neurological examination is normal.

Investigations

These are seldom required for a typical case.

Treatment

The condition usually resolves in 5–7 days, but persistence of symptoms beyond this time requires review of the patient and a questioning of the diagnosis. (The rare condition of rotatory subluxation of C1/C2 may present with features exactly the same as acute torticollis, but in this condition the pain and restriction of movement do not resolve.)

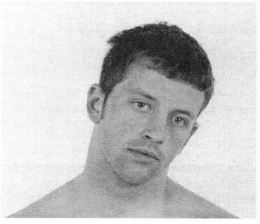

Fig. 15.5 • Acute torticollis.

Cervical spondylosis

Like any other joints in the body the cervical spine is subject to degenerative change. The joints (uncovertebral and facet) may develop osteophytes that may cause restriction in movement or compression of the nerve roots or the spinal cord.

History

The patient is often over 40 years of age. There may be a minor episode of trauma such as a fall, a blow to the head, or a minor road traffic accident. Pain and stiffness are the major symptoms. The pain is often poorly localized and may radiate anywhere from the interscapular area to the top of the head. Radiation to the shoulders is common, but radiation below the elbow should increase suspicion of root compression.

There may be a history of previous episodes. The patient is otherwise well. Ask specifically about lower limb symptoms.

Examination

Inspection is largely unremarkable. Palpation may locate a number of tender areas over the paraspinal muscles and trapezius. Movements are restricted, especially those of extension and rotation. Neurological examination is normal. *Any objective neurological sign requires a further opinion.*

Investigation

Normally not required for a typical case at initial presentation. The radiological changes do not appear to have a direct relationship to the degree of symptoms. Further investigation is required in those patients with atypical histories, prolonged severe symptoms, or neurological signs.

Treatment

This is largely symptomatic. The patient is encouraged to continue normal activity as much as possible. Simple analgesics are advised (the risk/benefits of NSAIDs in the older patient probably do not justify their use in this condition). The patient is referred to the GP for continuing care and review.

Patients with objective neurological signs, such as motor weakness or lost reflexes, should have an early review. *Any patient with lower limb signs or symptoms should be referred urgently.*

Referred pain

Pain from cardiac and lung disease may present in the neck. The combination of neck pain with no restriction in movement should raise the suspicion of referred pain. A very careful history and examination are required and further investigations such as ECG and CXR may be required.

Subarachnoid haemorrhage and meningitis cause neck pain, but headache is the major symptom.

Seropositive arthritis

The rheumatoid neck may give rise to acute problems such as subluxation of the odontoid. This may cause a sudden neurological deficit or signs of progressive long-tract compression.

Seronegative arthritis

Ankylosing spondylitis is an uncommon presentation in A&E medicine. The onset is often insidious and the diagnosis made by the patient's GP. As in rheumatoid arthritis, subluxations may cause cord or root compression.

These patients have a greater incidence of fractures or spinal cord damage even with minor trauma.

Other causes of neck pain

As in any other area, all the pathologies listed in 'softer tissues' may cause neck symptoms. Severe, atypical symptoms should be taken seriously and the patient referred for further follow-up either by the GP or an appropriate outpatient clinic.

Further reading

1. Bogduk, N. (1986). The anatomy and physiology of whiplash. *Clinical Biomechanics*, **1**, 92–101.
2. Fielding, J. W. and Hawkins, R. J. (1977). Atlanto-axial rotatory subluxation. *Journal of Bone and Joint Surgery*, **59-A**, 37–44.
3. Foreman, S. M. and Croft, A. C. (1988). Whiplash injuries. *The cervical acceleration/deceleration syndrome*. Williams & Wilkins, Baltimore.
4. Gargan, M. F. and Bannister, G. C. (1990). Long term prognosis of soft tissue injury of the neck. *Journal of Bone and Joint Surgery*, **72B**, 901–3.
5. McKinney, L. A. (1987). Early mobilisation and outcome in acute sprains of the neck. *British Medical Journal*, **299**, 1006–8.
6. Mealy K., Brennan H., Fenelon. (1986). Early mobilisation of acute whiplash injuries. *British Medical Journal*, **292**, 656–7.
7. Norris, S. H. and Watt, I. (1983). The prognosis of neck injuries resulting from rear end vehicle collisions. *Journal of Bone and Joint Surgery*, **65**, 608–11.
8. Pickin, M. (1995). A discussion of whiplash injury to the cervical spine. *The Journal of Orthopaedic Medicine*, **17**, 15–23.
9. Porterfield, J. and DeRosa, C. (1995). *Mechanical neck pain perspectives in functional anatomy*. W. B. Saunders, Philadelphia.
10. (Quebec Task Force) Spitzer, W. O., Skovron, M. L., Salmi, L. R., *et al.* (1995). Scientific monograph of the Quebec Task Force on Whiplash Associated Disorders: Redefining 'whiplash' and its management. *Spine*, **20–8S**, 1S–73S.

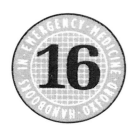

The back

Key points

- Sudden acute back pain is a valid reason for attending an A&E department.
- A full history and examination including neurological examination of the legs is essential.
- Examination of saddle area sensation and anal tone is essential.
- X-rays are not indicated in a young person after a lifting type of injury unless there are neurological signs or unusual features in the history.
- Neurological signs (severe bilateral limitation of SLR, bilateral motor/sensory loss, saddle anaesthesia/loss of bladder or anal tone) may indicate a surgical emergency — *refer.*
- Advice to mobilize, take analgesia, and to seek review by GP is given.
- X-ray is recommended in patients with significant trauma, the elderly, atypical history, prolonged symptoms, neurological signs.
- Referred pain from aortic aneurysm should be considered.

Thoracic spine injury

- Crush fractures common with minor trauma in the elderly.
- Crush fractures not uncommon in younger age groups even when only a moderate force is sustained.
- More severe forces tend to cause fractures at the cervicothoracic and thoracolumbar junctions.

Introduction

Back pain is very common. At some time in their life 58 per cent of the population will suffer from this condition. On any day of the year 14 per cent of the population will report back symptoms. There has been a shift in the treatment of this condition to preventive measures and self-management guidelines emphasizing gentle mobilization, exercise, and early return to normal function rather than a prescription for rest and adoption of the sick role.

The financial implications for the country due to days off work because of back pain reaches £3.8 billion. Sickness benefits cost £1.4 billion and the total NHS costs are £481 million with non-NHS costs (private consultations) being £197 million (CSAG report). Statistics also show that the longer the duration of sick leave due to an episode of back pain, the greater the difficulty in regaining full employment.

Approximately 6.9 million (16 per cent of the population) attend their GP per year with back pain. The A&Emergency department has also noted a large increase in the number of presentations with a figure of 480 000 per year in the UK (estimated cost of £17 million). There are many interactive factors that will determine the length of time an individual will be absent from work with a back injury, such as type of employment (self-employed people/short-contract workers have shorter absences), social status, psychological state, lifestyle, body composition, other illness, and nutrition.

There is a common misconception that patients with back pain are 'inappropriate attenders'. The 'mind set' that such patients are inappropriate may lead to less than adequate assessment and advice. Doctors often feel inadequate when faced with such problems, there is no 'magic bullet' that will guarantee cure. Acute back pain is an extremely painful condition and there is a small risk of serious pathology. While the majority of patients may be returned to the care of their GP it is essential to exclude problems such as spinal cord/cauda equina compression, and in the elderly tumour or pain radiating from an aortic aneurysm.

Anatomy

There are 12 thoracic and normally 5 lumbar vertebrae — sacralization of L5 or lumbarization of S1 may occur. The vertebrae articulate posteriorly at the facet joints (formed by the inferior articular processes of the higher vertebra and the superior articular processes of the lower) and by the intervertebral disc anteriorly. The orientation of the facets determines spinal movement and restricts most rotation in the lumbar spine.

The intervertebral disc is the equivalent of a 'shock absorber' as well as being crucial with its influence on the fluidity of movements in the spine.

The anterior longitudinal ligament is a major stabilizing structure attached to the anterolateral aspects of the vertebral bodies. Other ligaments are the interspinous, supraspinous, posterior longitudinal, and ligamentum flavum that help to stabilize the spine in flexion. The iliolumbar ligament connects the L5 transverse process with the ilium and is susceptible to injury in the flexed position.

Other supporting soft tissues are the fascial layers. The trunk muscles act as an internal corset to protect the back. These are the latissimus dorsi, erector spinae, serratus posterior, quadratus lumborum, the transversospinalis complex, plus the important abdominal muscle complex acting as antagonists and stabilizers (internal/external oblique and transversus abdominis).

The exact range of movement of the lumbar spine is difficult to measure clinically as thoracic spine and hip movements are involved in many of the classical methods of assessing lumbar spine movement; for example, bending forward to touch the toes since more than 50 per cent of this movement may take place at the hip joint. Commonly used measures of spinal movements are given below:

- flexion, increase in distance between T1 and S1 on full flexion from standing — 10 cm. Able to touch the floor or within 7 cm of the floor with fingertips;
- extension, 30 degrees (lumbar and thoracic);
- lateral flexion, 30 degrees;

* rotation, measured with patient sitting — 40 degrees (mostly thoracic).

The relationship of the spinal cord, cauda equina, nerve roots to the bony anatomy is summarized in Fig. 16.1. Note that the cord ends at the level of L1/L2. The lumbar and sacral roots continue distally and are at most risk of compression due to disc disease in the L3 to S1 area. The nerve roots leave the spinal canal via the intervertebral foramen whose boundaries include the disc and the intervertebral joints.

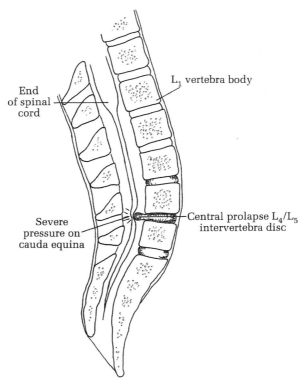

End of spinal cord

L$_1$ vertebra body

Severe pressure on cauda equina

Central prolapse L$_4$/L$_5$ intervertebra disc

Fig. 16.1 • Sagital section through the lumbar spine. Note the spinal cord ends at L1. The lumbar and sacral nerve roots (cauda equina) continue distally. Posterior protrusion of a lower lumbar disc may cause irreversible damage to these roots.

Radiation of pain

Back problems commonly cause pain to radiate to the legs. This can be of two types, true radiculopathy due to pressure on the nerve roots or damage to non-neural structures such as the dura, the intervertebral joints, and ligaments.

'Non-neural' pain is often poorly localized, does not follow any dermatomal pattern, and will usually not go below the knee.

True radiculopathy is less common, it follows a dermatomal distribution and the pain is worse with specific tests of neural stretch (sciatic and femoral stretch tests).

Examination

If the patient is able to walk, get off a couch, or out of a chair, then closely examine the movements to see if movement into lumbar flexion is carefully avoided.

Look

Standing. Observe for a scoliosis with the concavity of the lumbar spine towards or away from the pain. Unilateral muscle spasm of the erector spinae may also be present. Slow active movements into lumbar flexion, side bending, rotation, and extension should be assessed. Range of movement, pain on movement, and pain-limiting movement are noted.

Lying. Observe the patient getting into the lying position. As the patient is distracted, movements into lumbar flexion may suddenly become possible.

Feel — Gentle palpation of the lumbar spine is useful as any localized tenderness may point to a ligamentous rather than an annular pathology. Knowledge of surface anatomy will lead to palpation of the spinous processes, interligamentous structures,

-->

Fig. 16.2 ● Measuring spinal flexion. (A) Over 50 per cent of the movement in 'bending forwards to touch toes' occurs at the hips, shown here by keeping the spine straight with a stick. (B) A measure of true spinal flexion can be obtained by measuring the distance between the spines of T1 and S1 with the back extended. (C) The patient then flexes and the distance increases, in this picture shown by the gap between the end of the tapemeasure and the mark on S1.

sacroiliac joints, pelvic brim, lower costal margin, plus the deeper muscular and ligamentous soft tissues of the area. Guarding may also be a warning sign of a more sinister pathology.

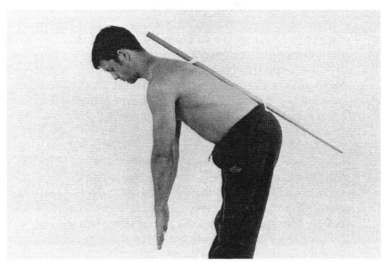

(A)

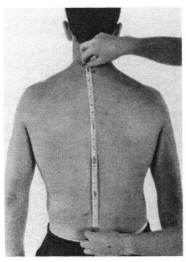

(B)

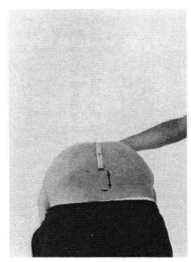

(C)

If pain allows, then also percuss the spinous processes (use the heel of your hand or a tendon hammer). The vertebral bodies are deep and pain may not be elicited by simple palpation of posterior structures.

Move — It may be difficult to isolate true lumbar movement. In bending down to touch the toes much of the movement comes from hip flexion, and thoracic spine movements also contribute (Figs 16.2A). However, the distance from the fingertips to the floor is often measured.

A better method to assess spinal flexion is to mark two vertebral spines (T1 and S1 for example). The patient then bends forward and the distance is re-measured. The expected increase in distance for the whole of the thoracic and lumbar spine is 10 cm (Figs 16.2B–C).

Lateral flexion is measured as is true rotation. Note that rotation is measured with the patient seated (Fig. 16.3). This movement takes place in the *thoracic spine*. Sometimes *simulated* rotation may be tested with the patient standing. In this movement the spine moves very little and severe pain on such movements might indicate an inappropriate response,

Passive movements of the spine may be tested in the sidelying position (Fig. 16.4). A mechanical problem in the spine will show restrictions on both active and passive movements, whereas in a mild disc lesion, passive movements may be free.

Function — Before, during, and after the examination the patient is observed as he/she walks into the room, moves around, gets on the couch, gets off the couch, gets dressed (e.g. can they put on shoes and socks with ease), sits, and stands. This observation may give important clues as to the severity of the pain.

Nerves and vessels — Neurological examination of the lower limb is essential. This should include power of quadriceps (L3/4), foot dorsiflexion, extensor hallucis longus (L5), foot

Fig. 16.3 ● Simulated and true rotation. (A) With the patient standing both the pelvis and the shoulders rotate, there is little or no spinal movement. (B) With the patient seated the pelvis is fixed. Rotation takes place in the thoracic spine.

plantarflexion (S1), knee flexion (S2/3). Sensation is examined
on the patella (L3), the big toe (L5), the heel (S1), and the back

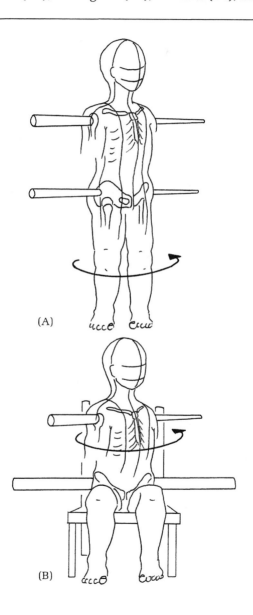

(A)

(B)

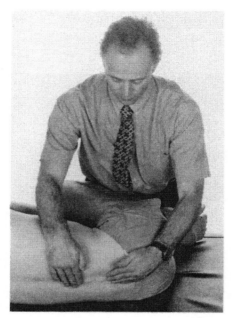

Fig. 16.4 ● Passive movement in side lying position.

of the leg (S2/3). The quadriceps, ankle, and plantar reflexes are examined.

The straight-leg raise test. A hand should also be placed under the hamstrings as tight musculature may mimic a positive test. Sciatic-nerve stretch tests may help confirm that limitation on straight-leg raising is due to pressure on the sciatic nerve (Fig. 16.5). In this test the limit of SLR is confirmed. The leg is brought back from this limit by 10 degrees. The ankle is then dorsiflexed, a movement that will stretch the sciatic nerve.

Abdominal examination may also be performed as pathology within this area may be the cause of back pain, e.g. aortic aneurism.

The saddle area sensation and the anal tone must be tested (Fig. 16.6). Failure to perform these tests will run the risk of missing a central-disc prolapse with cauda equina compression.

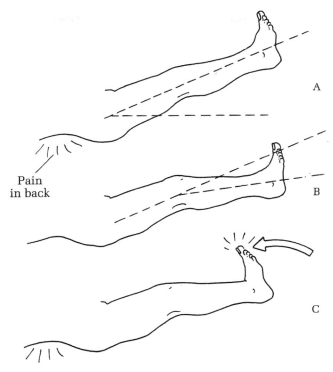

Fig. 16.5 • Sciatic nerve stretch test. (A) Straight-leg raise until pain is felt in the back. (B) Lower the leg until the back pain goes. (C) Dorsiflex the foot (stretches the sciatic nerve). If positive the back pain returns.

Trauma — acute back sprain

Introduction

This is the most common presentation. Most of these injuries will be due to ligament, muscle, or intervertebral joint damage (mechanical back pain). Some will be due to acute intervertebral-disc prolapse, although this will be the case in only a minority of patients. The prognosis is good with 90 per cent recovering from the acute attack within 6 weeks.

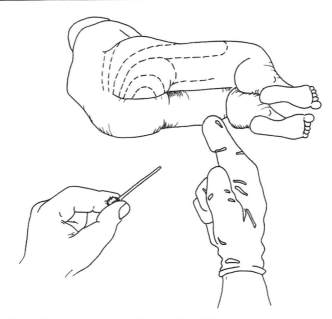

Fig. 16.6 ● Always check anal toe and saddle area sensation.

History

In the acute phase the pain is severe, the reason why the patient may present to A&E. The classic history is of the patient leaning forwards in a lumbar-flexed posture and then trying to lift a heavy object. As the weight is taken on there is a sudden, sharp, central back pain that causes the object to be dropped, the patient may fall to the floor or become 'locked' in the flexed position due to sudden muscle spasm (this occurs to limit the injury).

The other presentation with a similar, but milder, injury is of a sudden 'pop' sensation in the back followed by the development of pain several hours later as swelling and inflammation develops.

The pain in this acute phase may last for several minutes or hours and the patients only wants to lie down and stay still.

In a true prolapsed disc the pain is often worse in the leg than the back. Lumbar flexion, getting out of a chair, first thing in the morning (when the disc is more swollen), coughing, sneezing, and sitting can precipitate pain. The pain will usually radiate to the foot.

Relieving factors are lying down, gentle traction, and non-weight bearing exercises that have a soothing massage effect on the related musculature.

There is always the possibility of *spinal cord compression* presenting with neurology in the saddle area and loss of control of the bladder and bowel. *This is a surgical emergency and should be referred to the orthopaedic team on-call without delay.*

There are a number of factors in the history and examination that require a very full assessment and often referral (Box 16.1).

Examination

This is detailed above. Always check neurological function, the abdomen, and perianal sensation and tone.

Box 16.1 • Warning symptoms and signs in back pain

- Over 55 years of age
- Significant trauma (see below)
- Pain that is slowly getting worse, especially if night pain is a feature
- Weight loss
- Thoracic pain
- Past history of cancer, intravenous drug abuse, HIV infection, steroid usage
- Bilateral radiation of pain
- More than one myotome affected with progressive motor weakness or trouble walking
- Unable to pass urine/loss bowel control/saddle anaesthesia
- Associated abdominal pain

Investigation

In an acute back sprain X-rays will be normal. X-rays are not required at initial presentation in a young person (age 20–55) with a typical history, especially in young women. However, patients with an atypical history, the elderly, extreme pain, positive neurology, significant trauma (fall from more than 1 metre, road traffic accident, direct trauma), and any neurological findings should have X-rays. If the patient is not X-rayed then they should be reviewed by their GP, and if the pain is settling then X-rays should be considered (Clinical Standard Advisory Group report).

For a disc lesion with progressive neurological signs the investigation of choice would be an MRI scan, therefore refer to the orthopaedic team as a matter of urgency.

Treatment

If the patient can move, has no neurological signs, or no atypical history then he may be discharged home with the following advice:

1. Rest and take 48 hours off work if possible.
2. Take paracetamol for pain (or NSAID if no contraindications).
3. Start gentle exercises as soon as possible. For example, lay on your back, bend your knees and rock them from side to side. Start walking as soon as possible.
4. If symptoms continue then consult your doctor. Seek immediate medical advice if you have trouble in passing water or in controlling your bowels. **NB** Do not rest for more than 4 days. This will have harmful effects on your rate of recovery.
5. Stop smoking. Smoking delays the healing of damaged tissue.
6. If you are overweight then this is a good time to make a positive effort to lose some.
7. Swimming and static cycling are very beneficial if your pain is subsiding.

If the patient has difficulty with mobility then they may be sent home as long as there is responsible adult care for the patient. The elderly living alone may require admission for mobilization.

Provide analgesia and the advice sheet, plus a letter for the GP. The patient with neurological signs requires early follow-up by the GP as a minimum, but if there warning symptoms and signs then an orthopaedic opinion is needed. Progressive neurological signs and bladder or bowel disturbance require admission to hospital.

Significant trauma

This includes most falls over 1 metre, road traffic accidents (except minor rear-end collisions), and direct blows. Wedge fractures of the thoracic vertebral bodies are common in the elderly with minimal trauma, and even in the young and fit only moderate force may cause such injury.

The patient is likely to be brought in by ambulance, often immobilized.

The management should be along *Advanced Trauma Life Support Guidelines*. However, once life-threatening injury has been excluded then a detailed history of the mechanism of injury, symptoms and their progress, previous injury/illness are recorded.

Log-roll the patient. Examination may be limited to look and feel (percuss the spinous processes) and neurological examination until X-rays have been obtained. Obtain good quality films of the injured area. One common error is to ask for X-rays of the 'lumbar spine' or 'thoracic spine' when one of the most commonly injured areas is the thoracolumbar junction. Ask for views of the area of the spine with focal symptoms and tenderness.

Obtain orthopaedic advice if fractures are found or if there are neurological symptoms or signs.

Non-trauma — back pain

Sepsis

Infection in the gastrointestinal tract, gynaecological system, kidneys, and testicles may refer pain to the lower back. The history tends to be more suggestive of a visceral pathology and the abdominal examination may confirm this. Night pain may be the only symptom and sign of early osteomyelitis in the spine. Tuberculosis is returning to the differential diagnosis of infective causes of back pain.

Local sepsis may be a side-effect of local injection treatment or surgery. Fortunately, this is a rare problem.

Osteoarthritis

Degenerative change of the facet joints may be detected by restriction in active extension of the lumbar spine. X-ray and CT investigation may confirm this finding. Unless there is gross hypertrophy of the facets causing nerve-root or cord compression, then treatment is limited to gentle exercises and analgesia.

Spinal stenosis

causes bilateral leg pain (lateral canal stenosis causes unilateral symptoms) that becomes worse with exercise and is relieved by leaning forward. Altered sensation in the leg also occurs, and the symptoms and signs of spinal claudication require referral to the orthopaedic department as an outpatient for CT scan investigation of the spinal canal.

Fracture

Osteoporotic fractures, with no or minimal trauma, are common in the elderly. While these fractures are almost always treated conservatively, further follow-up is required to assess whether treatment is required for the osteoporosis and also to exclude more sinister diagnoses such as myeloma. If the vertebral body is severely crushed (more than 50 per cent) then seek orthopaedic advice.

Stress fractures

These occur in the lower back. The site most prone to stress injury is the pars interarticularis. The history is exacerbation of the pain with extension and rotation to the affected side.

Oblique X-rays and CT scans will detect the lesion. However, an isotope bone scan is a more sensitive test to detect an ongoing pathology. The use of MRI for the diagnosis of stress injury to bone is increasing in popularity, reliability, and sensitivity. Fractures at the pars will cause instability and chronic pain. Spondylosis and spondylolisthesis will occur.

Epiphyseal

Scheuermann's disease of the lower back occurs, but it is seldom the cause of the type of discomfort experienced in the thoracic spine (due to the different dynamics caused by a lordosis as compared with a kyphosis).

Referred pain

Referral of pain to the back may be due to pathology within the abdomen or pelvis. It is important not to miss the diagnosis of aortic aneurysm.

Tumour

The spine is a common site for metastases from the breast, prostate, thyroid, lung, kidney, bowel, testicle or deposits of multiple myeloma. The history is of an insidious onset of pain which is worse at night and disturbs sleep. Initial examination may reveal guarding and muscle spasm on palpating the spine. This muscular spasm/reaction is involuntary and totally different from the voluntary spasm produced by patients with hyperaesthesia associated with mild ligamentous inflammation. Further investigations for a primary cause will be carried out in the oncology department. The X-rays shows the moth-eaten appearance of osteolytic lesions or the sclerotic deposits that occur with prostatic carcinomata. In the early stages, however, plain X-ray may be normal and isotope scans may be required to make the diagnosis.

Other tumours are rare. A benign osteoid osteoma may cause few symptoms locally, but its size may cause referred pain. Aspirin apparently eases the ache caused by this tumour. It can be detected by a bone scan.

Pitfalls and how to avoid them

- *Cauda equina syndrome.* Perform a good neurological examination including the testing of saddle sensation and anal tone.
- *Missing fractures.* X-ray the elderly, those with significant trauma, and those with prolonged symptoms.
- *X-ray the appropriate part of the spine.* Especially where the tenderness is at the thoracolumbar junction, one of the commonest sites of severe spinal fracture.
- *Think of aortic aneurysm.* Remember this in the differential diagnosis of back pain.

Further reading

1. Bourdillon, J. F. (1990). The changing pattern of manual therapy. *Journal of Orthopaedic Medicine*, **12**, 3–5.
2. Bush, K. *et al.* (1992). The natural history of sciatica associated with disc pathology. *Spine*, **17**, 1205–12.
3. Clinical Standards Advisory Group Committee on back pain. (1994). *Back Pain*. HMSO, London.
4. Croft, P. *et al.* (1994). Low back pain in the community and in hospitals. *A report to the Clinical Standards Advisory Group of the Department of Health*. Prepared by the Arthritis and Rheumatism Council, Epidemiology Research Unit, Manchester.
5. Ellis, R. M. (1995). Back pain. *British Medical Journal*, **310**, 1220.
6. Hartman, L. (1985). *Handbook of osteopathic technique* (2nd ed). Hutchinson,
7. Hutson, M. A. (1990). *Sports injuries. Recognition and management*. Oxford University Press, Oxford.
8. Garoutte, B. (1981). *Survey of functional neuroanatomy*. Jones Medical Publications, California.
9. Jenner J. R., and Barry, M. (1995). Low back pain. *British Medical Journal*, **310**, 929–32.
10. McRae, R. (1990). *Clinical orthopaedic examination* (3rd Edn). Churchill Livingstone, Edinburgh.
11. RCS Working Party (1993). *Making the best use of a Department of Clinical Radiology. Guidelines for doctors* (2nd edn). Royal College of Radiologists, London.

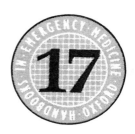

The chest

Key points

Blow to the chest

- In a patient presenting after a blow to the ribs perform a full respiratory examination.
- If the blow is to the lower ribs examine the abdomen.
- Perform a chest X-ray if there is any shortness of breath, raised respiratory rate, or chest signs.
- Those patients with chronic chest disease require extra care as the pain from a minor rib injury may precipitate respiratory failure.
- In a patient returning with chest problems after injury perform a chest X-ray.

Non-trauma

> **Be wary of diagnosing musculo-skeletal chest pain in a patient with no history of injury**

- **Death is not an infrequent complication of the misdiagnosis of musculo-skeletal chest pain — You have been warned!**
- Myocardial infarct, unstable angina, pulmonary embolus, pneumothorax, aortic aneurism, intra-abdominal problems should all be excluded.

Anatomy

The bony skeleton is made up of the 12 thoracic vertebrae, the ribs, costal cartilages, and the sternum. This bony cage protects the heart, lungs, great vessels, the liver, spleen, and upper abdominal organs (the abdomen reaches to the level of the nipple on inspiration). The intercostal vessels run close to the underside of the ribs. Tears in these vessels can result in a significant haemothorax.

Trauma — minor blow to chest

Bruised ribs, rib fractures, visceral injury

This is the commonest thoracic injury presenting to A&E departments, and while most of the injuries will be 'minor' they are often very painful. This section will only deal with minor injuries to the chest. A significant minority of patients with minor chest injury will develop immediate or delayed complications and full assessment is required. Those patients with an injury sustained in a road traffic accident or from a falls height over 1 metre require full assessment and a chest X-ray.

History

There is a history of a direct blow to the area, either during a fall, by an opponent in sport, or by an assailant. Determine the exact site of impact. This will raise the index of suspicion of damage to certain organs (e.g. the left lower ribs, the spleen, the posterior lower ribs, the kidney).

Often the patient will present 1–3 days after the injury, as the pain characteristically worsens over this period.

Ask the patient about any shortness of breath (distinct from pain on deep breathing), haemoptysis, other chest symptoms, and, if appropriate, haematuria or abdominal symptoms. Ask if the patient smokes or if there is a history of chronic respiratory disease.

Examination

Always measure the vital signs including respiratory rate (almost always forgotten). Determine the exact site of tenderness, and test for pain when compressing the chest at sites away from the area of the blow (e.g. pressing on the sternum and posterior ribs for an injury to the upper lateral rib area (Fig. 17.1). Pain on such compression indicates that there is a 'clinical fracture'. Examine chest expansion, percuss the chest, and listen to the breath sounds. Examine the abdomen in lower rib injuries.

Investigation

Have a low threshold for requesting a chest X-ray. If the blow is minor, the patient is well, there is no shortness of breath,

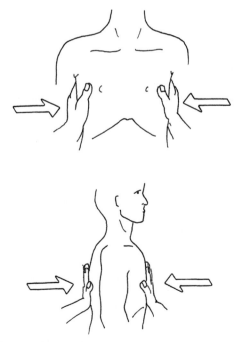

Fig. 17.1 • Chest springing for rib fracture.

and there are no abnormal signs in a patient with no previous chest problems, then a chest X-ray is not needed. If X-ray is not performed advise the patient to return if they experience increasing symptoms, especially shortness of breath.

Other investigations will depend on the clinical presentation, test the urine for blood in posterior injury, lumbar spine views may be required if the blow is to this area (transverse process fractures are relatively common), abdominal ultrasound to detect free peritoneal fluid may be required in lower lateral rib injury.

Treatment

'Minor' rib injuries are **very** painful. The pain stops the patient sleeping, moving normally, and involuntary splinting of the ribs causes localized hypoventilation. Give adequate analgesia (paracetamol/codeine preparations are traditionally prescribed, but opiates such an dihydrocodeine may be needed — use with caution in patients at risk of respiratory failure). Non-steroidal anti-inflammatory agents may be used in addition. Intercostal local anaesthetic blocks may give temporary respite, but are not routinely used in outpatients. Give patients advice to practice taking deep breaths for 5 minutes in every hour. Warn them that this will be painful, but that this can be helped by supporting the painful segment with a hand or pillow.

Even a young, fit individual can develop a chest infection due to hypoventilation. While it is not routine to prescribe prophylactic antibiotics, these should be considered in heavy smokers, and those with chronic chest disease. Older patients with chronic bronchitis and patients with poor respiratory reserve should be admitted to hospital if they have a rib fracture.

Advise the patient that if they develop respiratory symptoms (shortness of breath, purulent sputum, haemoptysis) they should return for further assessment. In a typical case with 1 or 2 rib fractures the pain is likely to be severe for 2 weeks and it will take 2 months to subside completely.

Complications

- pulmonary infection
- pneumothorax

- pulmonary contusion
- haemothorax
- empyema
- liver/spleen/kidney rupture.

Non-trauma

> **Beware the diagnosis of 'musculo-skeletal' pain in patients with no history of trauma**

General

It is true that many cases of non-traumatic chest pain are labelled 'musculo-skeletal' on inpatient discharge summaries. However, this is after investigation has excluded life-threatening diagnoses such as myocardial infarction, unstable angina, and pulmonary embolus. The inexperienced may include musculo-skeletal pain in the differential diagnosis, but should also consider the 'worst case scenario'.

History

This should be a full medical history noting all the features of the pain, associated symptoms, previous history, drug, family, and social history.

Examination

This must include recording of the vital signs and a general examination of the patient along with detailed examination of the chest, heart, abdomen, and legs (for signs of deep venous thrombosis). The finding of chest wall tenderness does **not** exclude more serious pathology.

Of all patients with acute myocardial infarction 15 per cent will have chest-wall tenderness.

Investigation

The investigation will depend on the clinical assessment, but ECG and chest X-ray are advised.

Treatment

Many patients will need admission. If the pain is typical of myocardial ischaemia then the provisional diagnosis must be either myocardial infarction or unstable angina, both require admission.

Other diagnoses

Sepsis

Any intrathoracic and intra-abdominal infections may present with chest pain.

Herpes zoster is common in the thoracic dermatomes, but may be difficult to diagnose before the onset of the rash.

Bornholm disease (infection with coxsackie B virus) must be one of the most common overdiagnosed conditions. It is a convenient label that is often applied to patients with chest-wall tenderness and signs of a systemic illness. While the disease may cause these signs it is prudent to think of all the possible diagnoses rather than 'latch on' to this label.

Osteoarthritis

Osteoarthritic changes are very common in the thoracic spine, but symptoms may be minimal even with severe radiological signs.

Costochondritis is an inflammation of the costochondral junction. This may occur after injury, but many cases are spontaneous in onset. To make the diagnosis there should be visible swelling of an isolated joint(s) with pain on compression testing (see Trauma — minor blow to chest). Treatment with a non-steroidal anti-inflammatory agent may be required.

Fractures

Crush fractures, 'cough' fractures, pathological fractures
Crush fractures of the thoracic vertebral bodies are common. In the elderly they may indicate osteoporosis or even osteomalacia. Treatment of the fracture is symptomatic with effective pain relief. The patient may require further investigation and perhaps treatment for any underlying problem such as osteoporosis. Such investigation is normally carried out by the patient's GP.

Referred pain

Dissecting aortic aneurysm, internal organs, abdomen, pleura, pneumothorax

The life-threatening nature of the differential diagnosis emphasizes the need for a thorough assessment of all patients with non-traumatic chest pain. The detailed diagnosis and treatment is outside the scope of this book, but the key to the diagnosis of these problems is to consider them in such patients.

Tumour

The thoracic spine and the ribs are prime sites for bony tumours. Myeloma should always be suspected in severe crush fractures. Secondary tumours are common in both the spine and the ribs. Spinal-cord compression is not uncommon in these patients, and a detailed lower-limb neurological examination should be carried out.

APPENDIX

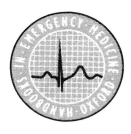
Musculo-skeletal problems — epidemiology and prevention

Epidemiology

Musculo-skeletal problems are the commonest reason for attendance at an A&E department. Reference to Table A3 shows that in a typical A&E department 36 per cent of patients attend with musculo-skeletal problems. Extrapolated to the whole country this would mean 3.5 to 4 million visits annually. Of these visits 75 per cent will be minor self-limiting problems, but 20 per cent will require some form of outpatient follow-up and 3 per cent will need emergency admission to hospital on their first attendance. The skill in managing musculo-skeletal problems lies in identifying those patients with more severe pathology who require more specific care or even admission. The magnitude of this task is shown in Table A1.

The distribution of musculo-skeletal problems around the body is summarized in Table A2. The hand and wrist, knee, ankle and foot account for 60 per cent of soft-tissue injuries. The distribution of non-traumatic musculo-skeletal problems is different with high rates of attendance for non-traumatic back and neck problems. There are also major variations in the rate of fractures in different areas. The large number of fractures of the hip is due almost entirely to fracture of the femoral neck in the elderly.

Causes of musculo-skeletal injuries

Table A3 shows the causes of musculo-skeletal problems presenting to an average A&E department.

Table A.1 • Numbers of patients presenting in 1 year with ankle problems to an average A&E department — 50 000 new patients per annum

Diagnosis	Number of patients
Simple ankle sprain	2200
Severe ankle sprain	260
Ankle fracture	470
Soft-tissue infection	160
Non-trauma	80
Tendon ruptures	5
Osteomyelitis	1 in 2–3 years

Table A.2 • Numbers of patients presenting with various musculo-skeletal problems to an average A&E department (50 000 new patients per annum). (The percentages apply to the body area in each row.)

Site	Numbers	Non-trauma (%)	# (%)	Admit (%)	Clinic (%)	X-ray (%)	Comment
Hand	4600	7	26	5.5	33	62	
Wrist	2400	6.4	47	7	50	81	
Forearm	900	13	20	13	25	51	
Neck	1200	23	2.5	6.3	5.5	55	42% RTA
Back	1000	32	8.7	10	3.1	43	
Ankle	3100	4.9	15	4.4	21.5	86	2200 sprains
Knee	2000	20	4.6	7.3	30	72	
Hip	600	16	44	54	6.5	90	#NOF

Table A.3 • Numbers of patients (rounded to nearest 50) with musculo-skeletal problems presenting to an average A&E department per annum

Cause	Numbers	Per cent of total musculo-skeletal problems
Falls	5800	34
Direct blow	2000	12
Sport	1500	9
RTA	900	5
Crush	750	4
Assault	750	4
Other injury	2300	13
Non-trauma	2000	12
Infection	1300	8
Total	17 300	

Simple falls account for most soft-tissue injuries seen in A&E practice. This comes from the **risk** that all humans have because of their upright posture with only two points of balance on the ground. Sport and road traffic accidents account for significant numbers of injuries. More detailed information on the exact causes of injury may may help the more effective targeting of accident prevention initiatives.

Prevention

Prevention is better than cure. A number of prevention measures have greatly reduced some types of musculo-skeletal injury. Seat-belt legislation greatly reduced the risks of serious injury following road traffic accidents. Paradoxically, it appears that this measure increased the incidence of one of the commonest minor musculo-skeletal injury, the 'whiplash' or neck sprain.

Apart from road and industrial safety there have been few scientific studies of injury prevention initiatives and much is left to common sense. Sport is one area where increasing emphasis is placed on prevention and this is discussed in detail below.

In the exercising population injuries are inevitable. However, this does not mean that they are acceptable. Advice can be given to treat acute injuries, self-management advice is also useful in preventing recurrent injury. An understanding of the biomechanics of sport and exercise is useful.

Self-management

Flexibility

This is an understated essential in the prevention of injury. If an athlete is expecting the body to respond to power demands, then the 'oiling of the engine' is required to prevent those demands becoming excessive. The more flexible a muscle, the more power can be generated. In contrast, tight, hypertonic muscle is far less efficient both physiologically and mechanically. Increased flexibility will allow a greater range of joint movement which is beneficial to performance.

Stretching prior to exercise is useful to warm-up the muscle, increase its blood supply, and inform the whole neuromuscular system of what is in store. Stretching after exercise has been shown to reduce postexercise soreness due to the resulting microtrauma.

Nutrition

Appropriate and adequate nutrition has to be understood and respected as the fuel that drives the x system. Dehydration is the main reason for poor performance and muscular cramps. During long-distance events a steady supply of carbohydrate is necessary. A 3-hour period should elapse after a meal before heavy exercise is undertaken. Poor nutrition may be present in the long-distance runner who is not replacing the not replacing the substrates being burnt up. Athletes who have to lose weight (judo, boxing) are susceptible to problems of dehydration.

Rest

Time and rest days are of great value in recovery from intensive training. Competing when tired is renowned for increasing the incidence of injury. It has been found in alpine skiing that 80 per cent of injuries occur in the final 2 hours of the skiing day.

Other measures

Attention to foot hygiene and nail care can prevent disabling conditions.

Sportswear

Clothing can cause injury such as skin-chaffing when wet. The use of substances such as Vaseline are indicated.

During events in hot temperatures, materials that are brief and breathe will allow the athlete to control his temperature by sweat evaporation.

In cold environments, a first layer of thermal clothing (that traps air and allows sweat to pass through) is covered by a second layer, such as cotton, that will absorb the sweat. The third layer should be wind-resistant with the final layer being of a waterproof nature.

Running shorts should be designed to prevent excessive movement of the scrotum and testicles and the development of joggers' testicle (haematoma of the epididymis).

Socks should be absorbent, and the shoes should give substantial shock absorbency, and support and be maintained in good order.

Sports equipment

Protective equipment

Face masks, protective boxes, gloves, shoulder pads, and helmets are mandatory in many sports and have been medically proven to prevent injury.

Other equipment

For example, the correct racket handle size and racket weight, the correct size of shoe, and the correct length of stud have to be taken into account to avoid persistent injuries.

Sports training

Overtraining is a common cause of injury. A sudden increase in the speed, duration, and/or intensity of training can be the cause of injury. Moving from a grassy to an artificial surface will obviously take its toll. Lack of respect for a new piece of equipment may also be to blame.

The athlete must avoid outdated coaching methods, such as running across a football pitch with an 82 kg man on your back. Training people the way that they were trained in the 1950s is not necessarily a good idea. Beware the traditionalist.

Sports assessment

A medical examination will highlight any contraindications to certain sports. Altered biomechanics of the foot is the cause of most bilateral lower-leg problems such as posterior tibialis tendinitis or patellofemoral pain brought on by exercise. Correct examination of the biomechanics of the foot during gait is a necessary dynamic assessment for a lesion that is undiagnosed on static examination. This is where video-analysis may be used. Treatment of these abnormalities is with corrective orthotics.

Further reading

1. Barrack, R. L. *et al.* (1989). Proprioception in the anterior cruciate deficient knee. *American Journal of Sports Medicine*, **17**, 1–6.
2. Hawkins, R. D. and Fuller, C. W. (1996). Risk assessment in professional football: an examination of accidents and incidents in the 1994 World Cup Finals. *British Journal of Sports Medicine*, **30**, 165–70.
3. Hutson, M. A. (1990). *Sports injuries recognition and management*. Oxford University Press, Oxford.
4. Maughan, R. J. *et al.* (1995). Dehydration and fluid replacement in sports. *Journal of Sports Exercise and Injury*, **1**, 148–53.
5. Renstrom, P. A. F. H. (1994). *Clinical practice of sports injury prevention and care*. Blackwell Scientific Publications, Oxford.
6. Ward, M. P., Milledge, J. S., and West, J. B. (1995). *High altitude medicine and physiology* (2nd edn). Chapman and Hall Medical,

Index

glenohumeral joint, *see* shoulder joint
gluteal tendinitis 189
golfer's elbow 125, 126
gout 68–9, 80, 83, 124, 144–5, 169–70, 223, 256, 257, 269–70
Group A streptococcal infections 54–5, 56

hallux 265–6, 269–70
hallux rigidus 269
hamate fractures 134, 138
hand 149–75, 320 Appendix
  anatomy 151, 152–3
  examination 153–8
  key points 151
  non-trauma 151
    pain and swelling in hand/finger 167–70
    pain in hand, no swelling 171–2
    sticking and clicking fingers/thumb 170
    weakness in hand 172–3
  pitfalls 173–4
  trauma 151
    bent finger back 153, 160–1
    bent thumb back/out 158–60
    crushed finger/hand 167
    dislocated finger 163
    finger will not bend/straighten 163–7
    'hit a wall' 161–3
    hit on end of finger 161
heat therapy 86
heel, pain under 272
herpes simplex virus 56
herpes zoster 56, 65, 317
herpetic stomatitis 56
herpetic whitlow 56, 167
hip and thigh 177–90
  anatomy and function 179
  examination 180
  key points 178
  non-trauma 178
    hip pain, adults 187–90
    limping child 182–7
    referred pain from 224, 273
  trauma 178
    direct/indirect to thigh 181–2
    hip pain after fall 180–1
history taking 12–15, 25–7, 28–9

hyperplantar flexion injury 254–5
hypertrophic pulmonary osteodystrophy 256
hypoventilation 315

ibuprofen 82–3
ice therapy 36, 46, 85–6, 251
iliolumbar ligament 296
infections, *see* sepsis
inferior tibiofibular joint 241
inflammatory phase 33, 34, 36–8
injection therapy 74, 83–5, 107, 108, 126, 170, 189
injury, *see* trauma
interferential 87
intermittent claudication 236
intracarpal joints 131
investigation
  non-trauma 28
  trauma 23–5
irritable hip 182, 185, 187
ischaemia 26, 28, 47, 66–7, 172, 190, 317
  and ankle pain 256, 257, 258, 259
  and foot pain 272, 273
  and leg pain 235–6
isokinetic testing 88
isometric testing 88
isotonic testing 88
isotope bone scans 60, 309

jogger's testicle 324 Appendix
joint above, examination of 16, 27
joint aspiration 28, 58, 205, 217, 223
joint replacements 58, 188, 221

Keinbock's disease 145
knee 21–2, 57, 191–224, 232, 320 Appendix
  anatomy and function 193, 194–7
  bony swelling 194
  effusions 194, 197–8, 214, 215, 217, 224
  examination 197–203
  functional giving way 194, 195, 218

WITHDRAWN
FROM STOCK
QMUL LIBRARY